Calculating and Reporting Healthcare Statistics

Fourth Edition

Loretta A. Horton, MEd, RHIA, FAHIMA

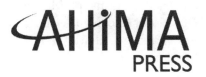

ISBN: 978-1-58426-317-313
AHIMA Product No.: AB120711

AHIMA Staff:
Jessica Block, MA, Assistant Editor
Claire Blondeau, MBA, Senior Editor
Adrienne Cook, JD, Developmental Editor
Katie Greenock, MS, Editorial and Production Coordinator
Ashley Sullivan, Project Editor
Jill S. Clark, MBA, RHIA, Reviewer

For more information, including updates, about AHIMA Press publications, visit http://www.ahima.org/publications/updates.aspx.

American Health Information Management Association
233 North Michigan Avenue, 21st Floor
Chicago, Illinois 60601-5809

ahima.org

Contents

About the Author

Loretta A. Horton, MEd, RHIA, FAHIMA, received a medical record technician certificate from Research Hospital and Medical Center and a bachelor's degree in psychology from Rockhurst College, both in Kansas City, MO; a health information administration post-baccalaureate certificate from Stephens College in Columbia, MO; and a master's degree in education, with an emphasis in curriculum and instruction, from Wichita State University in Wichita, KS. She also has completed graduate work in sociology at the University of Nebraska in Omaha.

Currently, Horton is co-chair of the Allied Health Department and coordinator of the Health Information Technology program at Hutchinson Community College in Hutchinson, KS. Previously, she worked in a variety of health information settings, including acute care and mental health, and has consulted with long-term care, mental retardation, home health, hospice, and prison systems. Additionally, she has worked as an instructor in the Health Information Administration program at The College of St. Mary in Omaha, NE, and for 3M as a marketing and training coordinator in Salt Lake City, UT.

Horton has been active in component state organizations as well as the American Health Information Management Association. She has served on the Item Writing Task Force for the Council on Certification, Council on Accreditation, and Scholarship Committee. She is a Fellow in the American Health Information Management Association.

Horton currently lives in Hutchinson, KS, with her husband, Bill, who is also a health information professional. She has two daughters, Merritt and Maura, and two grandchildren, Noah and Harriett.

Acknowledgments

Our thanks to Margaret Theodorakis, RHIT, CPC, CPC-H for her careful review of the text, exercises, and answer key for the fourth edition of *Calculating and Reporting Healthcare Statistics*, and for creating additional exercises to accompany the textbook.

A special word of thanks to Susan White, PhD, CHDA for her review of the text and insightful comments. Also, a word of thanks to the AHIMA Publications staff whose professional work helped to make this textbook a reality. A special thanks to Bill Horton, Becky Hageman, and Christopher Lau, who helped with a review of the textbook.

Chapter 1
Introduction to Health Statistics

Key Terms

Ambulatory care

Census

Descriptive statistics

Encounter

Home health (HH)

Hospice

Hospital

Inferential statistics

Inpatient

Inpatient census

Managed care organization (MCO)

Mean

Nursing facility

Outpatient

Primary data source

Research

Secondary data source

Visit

Vital statistics

Objectives

At the conclusion of this chapter, you should be able to:

- Define statistics

- Appreciate the need to study healthcare statistics

- Differentiate between descriptive and inferential statistics

- Recognize where statistics in healthcare originate

- Identify the users of healthcare statistics

Statistics

The term *statistic* refers to a number computed from a larger collection of numbers which collectively constitute a sample of data—for instance, the average value (or **mean**) of a variable belonging to a sample of data. A sample is a small part (a subset) of a larger group of data (a population). The term *statistics* is more broadly defined as a branch of mathematics concerned with collecting, organizing, summarizing, and analyzing data.

Origins of the Term

Originally, the term *statistics* referred to the collection of information about and for the "state." The word comes from the Italian word *stato,* meaning "state." One need only think of our own government and its statistics-collecting organizations, such as the Bureau of Labor Statistics, the National Center for Health Statistics (NCHS), the Administration on Aging, the Centers for Disease Control and Prevention (CDC), the Centers for Medicare and Medicaid Services (CMS), and so on.

Reasons for Studying Statistics

Statistics is really about decision making. In every area of our lives, we are expected to make decisions. To do that, we must have some information. Because information is often incomplete in healthcare settings, we must learn to estimate the characteristics of a complete population using statistics.

All organizations keep statistics in order to make decisions about their business. For example, an organization may use statistics to determine its markets, that is, to identify who is using its services and how it can increase those services. Libraries need information on what the public is reading in order to satisfy public interest and needs. Educational institutions need statistics about types of employment that students can get after graduation in order to improve the curriculum for future students.

Healthcare Operations Needs

In the healthcare industry, there are compelling reasons to collect and analyze data. For example, statistics kept on activities in the healthcare facility indicate why patients come to the facility and the costs of taking care of them. Patient care statistics and studies on performance can show the quality of care provided. Many accrediting agencies require a data analysis system as part of accreditation, and many third-party payers require facilities to collect performance data. Administrators also may use statistics for prioritizing needed services and to point to areas where efficiency and effectiveness might be increased. Additionally, healthcare facilities are interested in the types of patients they have with respect to their diagnoses in order to maintain the optimum physician specialty mix they need.

Public Health Needs

The government also needs to maintain statistics on and about the population in order to provide services. For example, the CDC is recognized as the lead agency responsible for protecting the health of the United States population by providing credible information to help individuals make the right healthcare decisions.

To obtain the knowledge they need, organizations first must have data. Data are unprocessed facts and figures that can be deliberately selected, processed, and organized to provide useful information. This leads, in turn, to facts, which are pieces of information representing the truth. And facts lead to an improved understanding of the original, unprocessed information. Improved understanding gives individuals the power to make better decisions. The sequence, then, is as follows:

Data → Information → Facts → Improved understanding → Better decision making

Health statistics provide information about the health of people and their utilization of healthcare services. Examples of healthcare statistics include average longevity, birth rates, death rates, incidence of a particular disease in a state or the United States as a whole, and the frequency of usage of a particular type of service within a hospital.

Other common uses of statistics may include divorce rates in a country, accident rates in a state, crime statistics in a city, percent of HIV carriers in the world, and even the standings of candidates in a political race. To serve each of these and many other purposes, the figures used in the statistics must be relevant and reliable. "To be relevant" refers to the applicability of the statistics. "To be reliable" means that there is some consistency of results. For example, if your instructor graded a test and then asked another instructor to grade the same test and they both had the same results, the results could be said to be reliable.

Descriptive Statistics versus Inferential Statistics

The primary focus of descriptive statistics is to organize and describe the features of data in a study. **Descriptive statistics** describe what the data show about the characteristics of a sample; in other words, they tell us information about a particular population. For example, we may need to know the average age of our patients or which service is used most in our facility. Both these statistics are used to describe data. **Inferential statistics,** on the other hand, help us make inferences or guess about a larger group of data by drawing conclusions from a small group of data. The smaller group of data is often called a sample, which is a portion of the larger group, or population. The results obtained from the sample, if gathered carefully, are assumed to be typical of the entire population.

Sources of Healthcare Statistics

Healthcare information is derived from both primary and secondary data sources. Statistics usually come from a primary data source, or firsthand documents. In healthcare, *primary data source* refers to the record that was developed by healthcare professionals in the process of providing care. *Secondary data sources* are data derived from primary sources. Secondary data sources are facility-specific. For example, the disease and operation index is a secondary source of information. All the information in the index comes from a primary data source—the health record. Registries are also considered secondary data sources. For example, information from the medical record may be used to create a cancer or trauma registry.

The health record is one of the most important primary sources of health statistics because it contains most of the health facts about patients.

Another source of health information is the census. A **census** is defined as a count of a particular population. The US government conducts a census, that is, a count of the people residing in the United States and their location. This kind of census is called a population census. "Census" comes from the Latin word *censere,* which means "to assess or to tax." The Romans started taking a census in order to make a register of the people and their property. One reason was to identify individuals who could serve in their armies and another was to place a value on their property so they could be taxed.

The US Constitution requires that a population census be taken every 10 years. The main reason is to determine the number of congressional representatives in the states. Over the years, Congress has authorized gathering more information about each person. The census now is used in many ways. For instance, the amount of government monies given to school districts is based partly on the number of children in a particular district. Congress also has requested that other types of censuses be taken periodically. These include a census of the types of businesses and industries in the US, for example, farms and fisheries, construction, foreign trade, manufacturing, and energy companies. All census information is available to the public.

Healthcare facilities also have a census, which is the count of patients present at a specific time and in a particular place. In **hospitals,** this is referred to as the **inpatient census.** The hospital census is a source of primary information. **Ambulatory care** facilities also may keep a census. This figure usually represents the number of **visits** or encounters during a specified period, usually one day. An **encounter** is defined in appendix B of this book as the direct personal contact between a patient and a physician or other person authorized by state licensure and, if applicable, by medical staff bylaws to order or furnish healthcare services for the diagnosis or treatment of the patient.

Hospital departments also keep statistics on the activities they perform for patients. For example, the laboratory department may keep data on the number of lab tests performed on **inpatients** and **outpatients.** The radiology department may keep track of the number of chest and hip x-rays. The physical therapy department may use statistical information such as the number of patient visits in deciding whether to hire additional physical therapists or add physical therapist assistants to their staff. These reports may be used in turn by the managers of the departments for productivity reports and combined to produce a report of activity for the entire facility. The administration of your hospital might ask you to keep data on the number of patients transferred to another hospital for a cardiac catheterization in order to determine the need for that service at your facility.

Another example of a primary source of information is **vital statistics.** The National Vital Statistics System (NVSS) is part of the National Center for Health Statistics (NCHS) of the CDC. These data are provided throughout the 50 states, Washington, DC, New York City, and five territories of the United States (Puerto Rico, the Virgin Islands, Guam, American Samoa, and the Commonwealth of the Northern Mariana Islands) to the NCHS. *Vital statistics* refers to a special group of statistics that record important events in our lives such as birth, marriage, death, divorce, and fetal death. Healthcare facilities are interested in births and deaths, fetal deaths, and induced terminations of pregnancy and generally are responsible for completing certificates for births, fetal deaths, abortions, and, occasionally, death certificates. All states have laws that require this information. The certificates are reported to the individual state registrars and maintained permanently.

The NCHS has developed standard certificates and procedures that states and territories must use to help facilitate the consistent collection of data. The standard certificates represent the minimum basic data set necessary for the collection and publication of comparable national, state, and local vital statistics data. The standard forms are revised about every 10 years, and the last revision was completed in 2003.

Data from the states and territories provide important information for use in medical research and are extremely valuable in estimating population growth in particular areas of the country and essential in planning and evaluating maternal and child health programs.

NCHS prepares and publishes national statistics based on vital statistics data because they are important in the fields of social welfare and public health. Because of their many uses, the data on these certificates must be complete and accurate.

Exercise 1.1

Identify the following as either a Primary Data Source or a Secondary Data Source:

Type of Healthcare Information	Source
1. Health insurance data pulled from national census	
2. Hospital census	
3. Productivity reports pulled from patient visit report	
4. Patient health record	
5. State vital statistics	
6. Tumor registry	
7. Hospital disease index	

Users of Health Statistics

All healthcare entities and third-party payers collect and use statistics. Following are examples of individuals and organizations that collect statistics and how they use statistics:

- Healthcare Administration: Inpatient facilities use health statistics to help address staffing issues and to determine the types of services to provide. For example, if the number of patients in the intensive care unit is increasing, the hospital administration may want to consider adding beds and staff to meet the growing need. Conversely, if a request is made to the hospital administration for new facilities and equipment that cannot be substantiated by the statistics, it is unlikely the request will be granted. Quality management departments in healthcare facilities collect data to determine how they are doing in regard to patient care and to how they can improve their patient care services.

- Healthcare Department Managers: Individual department managers in healthcare organizations use statistics to implement their department goals. For example, a manager needs to know if he or she is staying within budget. If not, the manager will need to investigate the reason.

- Cancer Registries: A cancer registry may be maintained by a separate department or may be a function of the health information department. States may also have a state cancer registry that is responsible for collecting data about cancer. A cancer registry collects data about the diagnosis, treatment, and follow-up of cancer patients. These statistics are important in tracking cancer survival rates. Facilities may choose to undergo accreditation through the American College of Surgeons. This is an evaluation by an independent team to determine whether the facility's cancer registry meets their standards. Statistics must show the facility is providing high-quality care and follow-up to its cancer patients.

- **Nursing Facilities:** Long-term care facilities may use statistics to determine the types of payers their patients have. These statistics also are helpful in demonstrating to the public the types of patients being cared for.

- **Home Health (HH):** Home health agencies provide care to elderly, disabled, and convalescent patients in their homes. These agencies keep statistics to determine the types of services used by their patients and their outcomes. For example, a home health agency would need to know the number of nursing visits, home health aide visits, physical therapy treatments, and patients with various types of equipment such as oxygen machines or other respiratory aids. Additionally, agencies will report patient outcomes, such as the number of patients who have improved, the number of patients who were compliant with taking their medications, or the number of patients who had to be readmitted to a hospital.

- **Hospice:** Hospice programs provide care and psychosocial support to terminally ill patients and their families. These services may be given in either the home or an inpatient setting. A hospice needs to know types of illnesses in order to match the appropriate caregiver with each patient.

- Mental Health Facilities: These may be inpatient or outpatient facilities. These facilities use health statistics to determine whether they are providing the proper services for patients in the community.

- Drug and Alcohol Facilities: These programs may be inpatient, ambulatory, or a combination of the two. Statistics are important in this area to show the success rates of these facilities' clients.

- Outpatient Facilities: These include physician clinics, surgery centers, emergency centers, and the like. Outpatient facilities often use statistics to determine whether they are providing the proper level of care to the community.

- **Managed Care Organizations (MCOs):** MCOs use statistics to determine whether they are providing the correct level of care at the best cost. Additionally, MCOs contract with healthcare facilities to provide specific services to their members at a particular cost. The MCO pays the agreed upon amount each time a member uses the service. Typically, the MCO receives a discounted rate and this results in individual members of the MCO paying less out of pocket.

- Healthcare Researchers: Researchers depend on healthcare statistics to perform **research.** Some examples include research in managed care, health law and regulations, mergers and acquisitions of healthcare facilities, physician practice issues, different types of illness and risk factors, telehealth issues, pharmaceutical research, and so on.

- Accreditation Agencies: These organizations use healthcare statistics to determine the most common diagnoses and procedures and whether the resources are available to treat patients with those diagnoses.

- Federal Government: The US government collects information for public health issues. For example, the CDC reports data on births, deaths, birth defects, cancer, and HIV/AIDS, just to name a few of the categories of data. CMS uses data collected by Quality Improvement Organizations (QIOs) for its quality improvement projects.

Handy Tip: Health information management (HIM) practitioners must remember that, first and foremost, statistics must be gathered and formulated, or expressed in systematic terms or concepts, before they even exist. HIM practitioners are usually the individuals who gather and formulate this information.

Because HIM practitioners have a broad knowledge of healthcare facilities as well as immediate access to a wide range of clinical data, they are in the best position to collect, prepare, analyze, and interpret healthcare data. HIM practitioners must learn acceptable terminology, definitions, and computational methodology if they are to provide the basic and most frequently used health statistics.

Chapter 1 Test

Select the best answer to the following questions:

1. In order to be useful, the figures used in statistics must be:
    a. fair and exact.
    b. relevant and reliable.
    c. honest and justified.
    d. simple and clear.

2. To be reliable, statistical information must:
    a. have some consistency.
    b. be applicable to what is being measured.
    c. be collected from one source only.
    d. have multiple meanings.

3. Descriptive statistics makes inferences or a best guess about a larger group of data by drawing conclusions from a smaller group of data.
    a. True
    b. False

4. Which of the following is NOT a primary source of statistics?
    a. Health record
    b. Vital statistics
    c. Hospital census
    d. Disease and operation index

(continued on next page)

Chapter 1 Test (continued)

5. What is the correct sequence to go from obtaining knowledge to use of that knowledge for decision making?

   a. Knowledge → Data → Information → Facts → Improved understanding → Better decision making
   b. Data → Information → Facts → Improved understanding → Better decision making
   c. Data → Information → Facts → Statistics → Improved understanding → Better decision making
   d. Information → Facts → Data → Improved understanding → Better decision making

6. The National Center for Health Statistics keeps statistics on:

   a. the licensing information on all healthcare providers in the 50 states.
   b. cancer and other deadly diseases in the 50 states and the US-owned six territories.
   c. vital statistics, such as births, deaths, and fetal deaths in North America.
   d. vital statistics, such as births, deaths, and fetal deaths in the 50 states and the US-owned territories.

7. Vital statistics are a primary data source for information.

   a. True
   b. False

8. Which user of statistics has the primary job of supporting terminally ill patients and their families?

   a. Home health agencies
   b. Nursing facilities
   c. Hospice
   d. MCOs

9. The CDC is the lead agency that:

   a. accredits and licenses acute hospital facilities in the United States.
   b. is responsible for providing vital statistics to various agencies, such as the NCHS.
   c. develops and updates ICD-10 for the world.
   d. is responsible for protecting the health of the people of the United States.

10. Which of the following is considered to be a primary source of information?

   a. The inpatient census
   b. Vital statistics collected by the NCHS
   c. The health record
   d. All of the above
   e. b and c only

Chapter 2
Mathematics Review

Key Terms

Average	Proportion
Decimal	Quotient
Denominator	Rate
Fraction	Ratio
Numerator	Rounding
Percentage	Whole number

Objectives

At the conclusion of this chapter, you should be able to:

- Explain fraction, quotient, decimal, ratio, proportion, rate, and percentage
- Understand the difference between a numerator and denominator
- Understand how to round whole numbers and decimals
- Convert fractions and decimals to percentages
- Understand how to average a group of numbers

Review of Basic Mathematical Expressions

Numbers may be expressed in a variety of ways for use in calculating statistics. The following sections discuss fractions, quotients, decimals, proportions, how to round numbers, percentages, ratios, rates, and averages.

Fractions

A **fraction** is one or more parts of the whole. Figure 2.1 shows two circles; the first circle is split into two equal parts, and the second shows one part of the circle larger than the other part. The fraction of the first circle is $\frac{1}{2}$; the fraction of the second circle (in darker color) is $\frac{3}{4}$. The top number is called the **numerator** and the bottom number is called the **denominator.**

> **Example:** Of the 40 patients with diabetes seen last month in a physician's clinic, 20 were Caucasian, 10 were African-American, and 10 were Asian-American. The following fractions show the number of patients of each race compared to the total number of patients who visited the clinic: Caucasian, $\frac{20}{40}$; African-American, $\frac{10}{40}$; and Asian-American, $\frac{10}{40}$. Fractions should be converted to their simplest form. Each fraction can be converted by dividing both top (numerator) and bottom (denominator) by a common factor. In this example, both the numerator and the denominator can be divided by 10: Caucasians, $\frac{2}{4}$; African-American, $\frac{1}{4}$; and Asian-American $\frac{1}{4}$. The first fraction can be further simplified with the common factor of 2; thus, $\frac{2}{4}$ can be expressed as $\frac{1}{2}$.

Exercise 2.1

Find the simplest form of each of the following fractions:

1. $\dfrac{40}{80}$

2. $\dfrac{3}{9}$

3. $\dfrac{75}{150}$

4. $\dfrac{6}{36}$

5. $\dfrac{20}{100}$

Quotient

A **quotient** is the number obtained by dividing the numerator of a fraction by the denominator. This number may be expressed in **decimals.**

> **Example:** The 14 members of your health information class decide to participate in your college's information day. The booth is going to be open for 21 hours over a three-day period. To find out how many hours each student would need to attend to the booth, you would divide the numerator (21 hours) by the denominator (14 students). This calculation gives a quotient of 1.5. Thus, each student would have to attend the booth for 1.5 hours.

Figure 2.1. 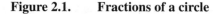   **Fractions of a circle**

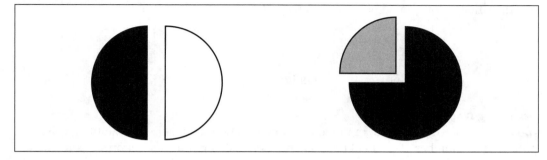

Decimal Fraction

Decimal fractions are simply referred to as decimals. The notation indicates a value that is less than one. In 14.37, for example, the digits to the right of the decimal point (3 and 7) are called decimal digits. The decimal point is used to separate the fraction of a **whole number** (.37) from the whole number itself (14). The decimal point is not ordinarily used in whole numbers (for example, 14.0) unless the healthcare facility has a particular reason for doing so.

> **Handy Tip:** The decimal .5 is usually written as 0.5 in order to call attention to the decimal point.

Rounding Numbers

Rounding is a process of approximating a number. Numbers may be rounded to the nearest 10, 100, and so on.

Rounding to the Nearest Ten

Rounding to the nearest ten means that any number between multiples of ten (10, 20, 30, 40, and so on) is rounded to the multiple it is closest to. For example, 31 falls between 30 and 40 but is closer to 30, so it is rounded to 30. However, 37 is closer to 40, so it is rounded to 40. When a number is exactly between the two multiples of ten, the rule of thumb is to round up. Thus, the 5 in the ones place indicates 35 would be rounded up to 40 as in the example below.

$$
\begin{array}{cc}
3 & 5 \\
\downarrow & \downarrow \\
\text{tens} & \text{ones}
\end{array}
$$

Rounding to the Nearest Hundred

Rounding to the nearest hundred refers to rounding numbers that fall between multiples of 100. For example, 327 falls between 300 and 400 but is closer to 300. Thus, the 2 in the tens place indicates that 327 should be rounded down to 300.

$$
\begin{array}{ccc}
3 & 2 & 7 \\
\downarrow & \downarrow & \downarrow \\
\text{hundreds} & \text{tens} & \text{ones}
\end{array}
$$

The number 7,868 falls between 7,800 and 7,900. In this case, the 6 (in the tens place) indicates that 7,868 should be rounded up to 7,900.

7	8	6	8
↓	↓	↓	↓
thousands	hundreds	tens	ones

Rounding Decimals

Most healthcare statistics are reported as decimals, and each healthcare facility has its own policy on the number of decimal places to be used in computing and reporting percentages. The principles that apply to rounding whole numbers also apply to rounding decimals. To round to the nearest whole number, look at the first digit to the right of the decimal point (tenths); if the number is 5 or more, the whole number should be rounded up; if the number is less than 5, the whole number should be left as it is. Thus, the whole number in 14.4 should remain at 14; however, 14.5 should be rounded up to 15.

To round to the nearest tenth, you do the same thing except use the hundredths digit rather than the tenths. The hundredths is the second digit to the right of the decimal point. For example, 14.46 would be rounded up one to 14.5 because the 6 in .46 is greater than 5. In the case of 14.13, the 3 in .13 is less than 5, so the .1 is kept rather than rounding up. To round to the nearest hundredths, the calculation must be carried out to three decimal places (the thousandths digit) and then rounded. For example, 14.657 would be rounded up to 14.66 because the 7 in .657 is greater than 5. In the case of 14.654, the 4 in .654 is less than 5, therefore the decimal is rounded down to 14.65.

Handy Tip: When the decimal points must be carried out to two places, the calculation should be carried out to one more place in the quotient and rounded back. For example:

$$\frac{1}{7} = 0.142 = 0.14$$

Exercise 2.2

Find the quotient in the following fractions. Round to two decimal places.

1. $\frac{3}{5}$
2. $\frac{8}{12}$
3. $\frac{34}{56}$
4. $\frac{107}{98}$
5. $\frac{545}{654}$

Exercise 2.3

Round the following numbers to the nearest 10.

1. 48
2. 356
3. 311
4. 5,896
5. 3,258
6. 9,631
7. 232,563
8. 2,634
9. 48,605
10. 8,563

Round the following numbers to the nearest hundred.

11. 651
12. 123
13. 8,307
14. 7,534
15. 5,781

Round to the nearest whole number.

16. 18.3
17. 32.5
18. 23.1
19. 152.6
20. 99.4

Round to one decimal place.

21. 15.89
22. 18.58
23. 32.62
24. 99.98
25. 124.07

(continued on next page)

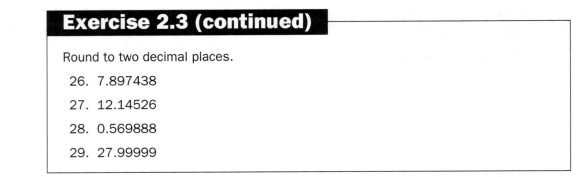

Exercise 2.3 (continued)

Round to two decimal places.

26. 7.897438

27. 12.14526

28. 0.569888

29. 27.99999

Percentage

The ratio of a part to the whole is often expressed as a **percentage.** A percentage is a fraction expressed in hundredths. Percent means "per 100." There is a specific way to write this. For example, .34 would be written as $\frac{34}{100}$ and is equal to 34 percent.

Percentages are a useful way to make fair comparisons. For example, if 20 patients died in hospital A last month and 50 patients died in hospital B during the same period, one might conclude that it would be better to use the services at hospital A because hospital A had fewer deaths. However, that conclusion would be wrong if hospital A had 100 discharges during the month and hospital B had 500 discharges for the same period.

Hospital A: 20/100 = 20%
Hospital B: 50/500 = 10%

Not all percentages are converted to whole numbers. For example:

$$\frac{1}{8} = .125 = 12.5\%$$

Changing a Fraction to a Percentage

To change a fraction to a percentage, divide the numerator by the denominator and multiply by 100. For example, to change $\frac{1}{2}$ to a percentage, divide 1 by 2 and multiply by 100. The calculation is as follows:

$$\frac{1}{2} = 0.5 \times 100 = 50\%$$

Changing a Decimal to a Percentage

To change a decimal to a percentage, simply multiply the decimal by 100. The calculation changes the position of the decimal point. For example:

$$0.29 \times 100 = 29\%$$

Changing a Percentage to a Fraction

To convert a percentage to a fraction, eliminate the percent sign and multiply the number by $\frac{1}{100}$. A simpler version of this is to place the number in the numerator and 100 in the denominator. For example:

$$5\% \text{ would be } 5 \times \frac{1}{100} = \frac{5}{100}$$

$$15\% \text{ would be } 15 \times \frac{1}{100} = \frac{15}{100}$$

Fractions are usually converted to their simplest form. In the example of 5 percent, both 5 and 100 can be divided by 5, which would result in a fraction of $\frac{1}{20}$. In the example 15 percent, again, both 15 and 100 are divisible by 5, resulting in a fraction of $\frac{3}{20}$.

Changing a Percentage to a Decimal

To convert a percentage to a decimal, eliminate the percent sign and place a decimal point two places to the left. If the percentage is only one digit, place a 0 in front of it and place the decimal point in front of the 0. For example:

76 percent would be 0.76

4 percent would be 0.04

104 percent would be 1.04

Exercise 2.4

Complete the following conversions.

Fractions to percentages (round to one decimal place):

1. $\frac{3}{4}$

2. $\frac{4}{5}$

3. $\frac{7}{8}$

4. $\frac{9}{10}$

5. $\frac{1}{15}$

Decimals to percentages:

6. 0.75

7. 0.09

8. 0.16

9. 0.325

10. 0.965

Percentages to fractions:

11. 35%

12. 82%

13. 25%

14. 4%

15. 33%

(continued on next page)

Exercise 2.4 (continued)

Percentages to decimals:

16. 17%

17. 3%

18. 0.5%

19. 118%

20. 99%

21. A pediatrician in your local physician's clinic saw 50 children in one week for their preventive well-baby checkup. 32 received the MMR vaccine.

    Express the rate of the MMR administration in percent. Round to one decimal place.

22. During the year 2005, there were 884,974 physicians of various specialties in the United States. The following specialties made up a part of that figure. Using the information below, what percentage of the whole did these specialties make up? Round to two decimal places.

    - Forensic Pathologists   620
    - Medical Genetics   476
    - Ophthalmologists   18,706
    - Internal Medicine   150,933

23. The physician practice you work for needs a new shredder. They want a cross-cut shredder that can cut 20 sheets at a time. It must be strong enough to destroy staples and small paper clips with a waste bin of at least eight gallons. You did some investigation and secured five offers from different companies. The shredders are all of equal quality. Using the information below, which company is giving you the best deal?

	List Price	Discount	Cost of Two-Year Replacement Warranty	Shipping and Handling	TOTAL COST
Company A	$579.00	20%	$20.00	Local $00.00	
Company B	$625.00	30%	$25.00	$25.00	
Company C	$600.00	20%	$20.00	Free $00.00	
Company D	$551.00	15%	$18.00	$33.00	
Company E	$584.00	25%	$25.00	$30.00	

Exercise 2.5

Using the information found in the scenario below, answer the following questions.

Forty patients were seen in the Hematology/Oncology Clinic last Tuesday. Twenty patients had sickle-cell anemia, twelve patients had hemophilia, six patients had Ewing's sarcoma and two had Wilms' tumor.

1. Express in fractions the number of patients with each condition compared to the number of patients who visited the clinic last Tuesday. Remember to convert each fraction to its simplest form.

Sickle-Cell	Hemophilia	Ewing's Sarcoma	Wilms' Tumor

2. Express in decimals the number of patients with each condition compared to the number of patients who visited the clinic last Tuesday.

Sickle-Cell	Hemophilia	Ewing's Sarcoma	Wilms' Tumor

3. Express in percents the number of patients with each condition compared to the number of patients who visited the clinic last Tuesday.

Sickle-Cell	Hemophilia	Ewing's Sarcoma	Wilms' Tumor

Ratio

Three general classes of mathematical parameters are used to relate the number of cases, diseases, patients, or outcomes in the healthcare environment to the size of the source population in which they occur. The most basic measure is the **ratio**. A ratio expresses the relationship of one quantity to another.

Calculating Ratio

To calculate a ratio, one quantity is divided by another. The number can be greater than 1 or less than 1. For example, if seven men and five women were in a group, the ratio of men to women would be $\frac{7}{5}$. This ratio also may be written as 7:5 and verbalized as 7 to 5. The numbers 7 and 5 have no common factors, so this ratio cannot be simplified. However, if the group consisted of 6 men and 10 women, for example, the ratio would be 6:10. Because the numbers in this ratio have a common factor of 2, the ratio can be simplified by dividing each number by 2, which simplifies the ratio to 3:5. This is done the same as before in the section on fractions. This is converted by dividing both the top and bottom numbers by a common factor. In this example, both numbers can be divided by 2.

$$\text{Ratio} = \frac{x}{y} = \frac{6}{10} = \frac{\frac{6}{2} = 3}{\frac{10}{2} = 5}$$

or

$$\text{Ratio} = \frac{y}{x} = \frac{10}{6} = \frac{\frac{10}{2} = 5}{\frac{6}{2} = 3}$$

Exercise 2.6

Express the following ratios in their simplest form.

1. 14:28
2. 3:12
3. 5:10
4. 7:49
5. 1:16
6. A group of 12 men and 18 women have diabetes. Express the ratio of men with diabetes to women with diabetes. Calculate it to its simplest form.

Proportion

A **proportion** is a type of ratio in which x is a portion of the whole $(x + y)$. In a proportion, the numerator is always included in the denominator. For example, if two women out of a group of 10 over the age of 50 have had breast cancer, where $x = 2$ (women who have had breast cancer) and $y = 8$ (women who have not had breast cancer), the calculation would be 2 divided by 10. The proportion of women who have had breast cancer is 0.2.

$$\frac{x}{(x + y)} = \frac{2}{(2 + 8)} = 0.2$$

Exercise 2.7

1. A school district wants to know the proportion of students who have deferrals for mandated vaccines. School #2 has 450 students. Of the 450 students, 435 students are up to date on their vaccines. There are 15 students with deferrals. What is the proportion of students with deferrals who have not been vaccinated? Round to two decimal places.

2. In a group of 50 persons, 12 have Type II diabetes mellitus.

   What is the proportion of people in the group that have diabetes? Express as a decimal and round to two decimal places.

Rate

A **rate** is a ratio in which there is a distinct relationship between the numerator and denominator and the denominator often implies a large base population. A measure of time is often an intrinsic part of the denominator. Healthcare facilities calculate many types of rates in order to determine how the facilities are performing.

> **Handy Tip:** Misplaced decimal points can result in mathematical errors. All calculations should be checked for sensible answers. For example, a hospital death rate of 25 percent should seem unreasonable because it indicates that one of every four patients treated at this hospital died. Why would anyone want to be treated at a hospital that had a 25 percent death rate? Thus, the decimal placement in this calculation should be checked. The correct death rate for this hospital may be 2.5 percent or 0.25 percent, which would be more realistic.

The term *rate* is often used loosely to refer to rate, proportion, percentage, and ratio. Indeed, many books and organizations use these terms interchangeably. For this reason, it is important to be aware of how any measure being reported has actually been defined and calculated.

Calculating Rate

The basic rule of thumb for calculating rate is to indicate the number of times something *actually* happened in relation to the number of times it *could have* happened (actual/potential). For example, let's say you have been eating out often in the past few weeks. To calculate the rate of meals you have eaten out in one week, divide the number of meals that you ate out (for example, 13) by the number of meals you could have eaten out (21). The rate is $\frac{13}{21}$, or 61.9 percent. The formula for determining rate is as follows:

$$Rate = \frac{Part}{Base}, \text{ or } R = \frac{P}{B}$$

Table 2.1 shows the equations for calculating ratio, proportion, percentage, and rate.

Table 2.2 shows a sample computerized statistical report provided by the information systems (IS) department of an acute care facility and illustrates how the department uses percentages.

> **Handy Tip:** Everyone has heard this saying about computers: "garbage in, garbage out," or "GIGO." Computers are great for many things, including performing statistical calculations, but they must be programmed accurately to calculate correctly. Even the function of rounding needs to be validated.

Table 2.1.   Review of equations for calculating ratio, proportion, percentage, and rate

The following list of equations differentiates among ratio, proportion, percentage, and rate, where $x = 5$ men and $y = 3$ women.

Ratio: $\dfrac{x}{y} = \dfrac{5}{3}$

Proportion: $\dfrac{x}{(x + y)} = \dfrac{5}{(5 + 3)}$

Percentage: $\left[\dfrac{x}{(x + y)}\right] \times 100 = \left[\dfrac{5}{(5 + 3)}\right] \times 100$

Rate: $R = \dfrac{Part}{Base}$ or $R = \dfrac{P}{B}$

Table 2.2.   Administrator's semiannual reference report

Administrator's Semiannual Reference Report Admissions by Day of Week 1/1/20XX–6/30/20XX		
Day	**Number of Patients**	**Percent of Patients**
Sunday	1,187	19.1
Monday	755	11.3
Tuesday	1,085	16.3
Wednesday	1,031	15.5
Thursday	1,024	17.0
Friday	808	12.1
Saturday	773	11.6
Total	**6,663**	**100.0**

For example, it is not unheard of for an IS manager to ask a health information management (HIM) professional for the formula for death rate because the computer system crashed and all new formulas and specifications had to be reprogrammed.

Averages

An **average** is the value obtained by dividing the sum of a set of numbers by the number of values. Average is generally referred to as the arithmetic mean to distinguish it from the mode or median. (This is covered in more detail in chapter 10.)

The symbol $\overline{X}$ (pronounced "ex bar") is used to represent the mean in this formula.

$$\frac{Sum\ of\ all\ the\ values}{Number\ of\ all\ the\ values\ involved} = \overline{X}$$

Example: Let's say that you have taken six medical terminology tests. Your scores are 82, 78, 94, 56, 91, and 85. Adding together the scores gives you a total score of 486. Now, divide this by 6 (the number of tests you have taken). This equals 81. This means that your average score on the medical terminology tests is 81.

Exercise 2.8

The following were the recorded birth weights for babies born Jan. 22, 20XX: 5.5 lbs, 5.0 lbs, 7.7 lbs, 8.9 lbs, 4.6 lbs, 7.3 lbs, 6.5 lbs, 6.8 lbs, 8.0 lbs, and 8.13 lbs.

What was the average birth weight for the day? Round to two decimal places.

Chapter 2 Test

Complete the following exercises.

1. Convert the fraction $\frac{1}{5}$ to a quotient and then a percentage.

Chapter 2 Test (continued)

2. Round the following percentages to two decimal places.

   a. 15.894%
   b. 13.256%
   c. 0.765%
   d. 0.068%
   e. 56.325%

3. Convert $\frac{1}{6}$ to a percentage to two decimal points.

4. Review table 2.2 to verify that the calculations are correct. Note that the percent of patients listed in this report is the actual/potential.

$$\left(\frac{\textit{Actual \# of patients}}{\textit{Potential \# of patients}} \right) \times 100$$

5. It was reported in your department meeting that over the past year your hospital increased the number of employees by 12 percent. Last year there were 347 people employed; how many are employed this year? (Round to a whole number.)

6. Your manager needs to purchase a personal computer for the new receptionist in your department. The usual price is $1,100. The local supply company gives the facility an 11.5 percent reduction on all items they purchase. What price will your manager pay?

7. Your beginning salary as an analyst in the HIM department is $12.50 per hour. You are due to receive a 3.5 percent cost-of-living raise in your next paycheck. Your performance evaluation is coming up in one month, and you believe you should get an additional 4 percent increase based on your excellent performance. What should your hourly wage be after your next paycheck, and what do you anticipate it will be after your performance evaluation?

8. Last year, you purchased equipment in the HIM department for $10,250. You have been told that the equipment you bought has depreciated in value by 15 percent. What is the value of the equipment now?

9. You just scored 15 correct out of a possible 40 on your health information test. What percentage did you earn?

10. Last year, the number of hospitals in your state decreased from 320 to 240. What is the percentage of decrease?

11. During the last week Community Hospital reported that the following numbers of patients were discharged:

    Sunday—18; Monday—22; Tuesday—37; Wednesday—25; Thursday—22; Friday—28; Saturday—12

    What is the average number of patients discharged during the week? (Round to a whole number.)

For the following questions, refer to the Quarterly Coder Accuracy Report on the next page.

12. Are the calculations of the percentage of records accurately coded for each month and the total for the quarter correct?

13. Coder D determined her accuracy rate for the quarter to be 95.9 percent. She would like you to recalculate her accuracy rate because she thinks it is incorrect in the report.

(continued on next page)

Chapter 2 Test (continued)

Community Hospital
Quarterly Coder Accuracy Report
January–March 20XX

	January			February			March			Total		
	# Records	# Correct	% Correct	# Records	# Correct	% Correct	# Records	# Correct	% Correct	# Records	# Correct	% Correct
Coder A	560	504	90.0%	544	495	91.0%	270	243	90.0%	1,374	1,242	90.4%
Coder B	540	503	93.1%	523	491	93.9%	531	494	93.0%	1,594	1,488	93.4%
Coder C	500	440	88.0%	445	401	90.1%	493	435	88.2%	1,438	1,276	88.7%
Coder D	620	583	94.0%	588	570	96.9%	584	551	94.3%	1,792	1,704	95.1%
Coder E	480	408	85.0%	432	392	90.7%	465	397	85.4%	1,377	1,197	86.9%
Total	**2,700**	**2,438**	**90.3%**	**2,532**	**2,349**	**92.8%**	**2,343**	**2,120**	**90.5%**	**7,575**	**6,907**	**91.2%**

Chapter 3
Patient Census Data

Key Terms

Average daily inpatient census

Calculation of inpatient service days

Calculation of transfers

Census day

Complete master census

Daily inpatient census

Hospitalization

Inpatient admission

Inpatient census

Inpatient service day

Intrahospital transfer

Leave of absence

Patient care unit (PCU)

Patient day

Recapitulation

Total inpatient service days

Objectives

At the conclusion of this chapter, you should be able to:

- Define, differentiate, and apply the terms inpatient census, daily inpatient census, inpatient service day, total inpatient service days, and admission and discharge (A&D)

- Differentiate between an interhospital (interfacility) transfer and an intrahospital transfer

- Compute daily census and inpatient service days using the admission and discharge data provided

- Compute census and inpatient service days with data given for births and transfers

- Compute the average daily inpatient census for a patient care unit given inpatient service days for any such unit

Inpatient Census

Hospital management uses census data for various purposes, including planning, budgeting, and staffing. The **inpatient census** indicates the number of patients present in the healthcare facility at a particular point in time. Hospitals include only inpatients in their calculations.

An individual on each **patient care unit (PCU)** is designated to count the patients on that unit each day. The inpatient census-taking time is usually at midnight but may occur at any time as long as the time is consistent for the entire facility, that is, each PCU conducts the census at the same time. Around midnight is actually a good time to take the census because patients are usually in their beds. It would be difficult to account for all patients at 8:00 a.m., for example, because they might not be in their beds. They may be in exam rooms, radiology, surgery, with their healthcare provider, or just taking a walk in the hospital.

In a manual system, the census taker fills out a form to be sent to a central collection area (usually the nursing office, information systems, admissions, health information department, or any other office designated by the administration). The names of patients admitted, discharged, and transferred to or from a PCU appear on the form. This makes it easier for the central collection area to discover any discrepancies in the data from the PCUs and to know where each patient is located at all times.

In a computerized system, the necessary data are first entered into the computer as admissions, discharges, or transfers and then verified at the designated time by the responsible person on each PCU.

Handy Tip: A PCU is an organizational entity of a healthcare facility such as a medicine unit, surgery unit, or special unit such as the intensive care unit (ICU) or cardiac care unit (CCU). This should not be confused with medical services, which refer to the activities relating to medical care performed by physicians, nurses, and other healthcare professionals and technical personnel under the direction of a physician.

Table 3.1 shows a form for a manual daily census summary for a nursing home.

Complete Master Census

In addition to reporting the head count to the central collection area, each PCU reports, in written form or via computer, the number of patients admitted, discharged, and transferred in or out that day. This is commonly referred to as the ADT system in a facility. The central collection area then uses the census from all the units to compile a total census for the facility, sometimes referred to as the **complete master census.** The complete master census shows the names of patients present at a particular point in time and their location. In most facilities this is a computerized process that is linked with the facility's master patient index, billing system, and other electronic health record systems.

Handy Tip: In this book, the term *transfer* in a hospital setting refers to an intrahospital transfer. **Intrahospital transfers** are patients who are moved from one PCU to another within the facility. The transfers in and transfers out on an individual PCU may not be equal because it is possible to transfer more patients in than transfer out and vice versa. However, the total intrahospital transfers in must always equal the intrahospital transfers out.

Table 3.1.   Daily census summary at Community Manor Nursing Home

To be completed daily at 12:01 a.m. by charge nurse			Community Manor Nursing Home Daily Census Summary	
Hall: ____A ____B ____C ____D			**Date** _____	
Initial admits—New residents			Date	Time
				a.m.–p.m.
				a.m.–p.m.
				a.m.–p.m.
				a.m.–p.m.
Discharged to home or transfer			Date	Time
				a.m.–p.m.
				a.m.–p.m.
				a.m.–p.m.
Transfer to hospital	Location		Date	Time
				a.m.–p.m.
				a.m.–p.m.
				a.m.–p.m.
				a.m.–p.m.
Out on leave—Pass	Date Left	Time	Returned	Time
		a.m.–p.m.		a.m.–p.m.
		a.m.–p.m.		a.m.–p.m.
		a.m.–p.m.		a.m.–p.m.
Deceased			Date	Time of Death
				a.m.–p.m.
				a.m.–p.m.
				a.m.–p.m.
Return from hospital stay			Date	Time
				a.m.–p.m.
				a.m.–p.m.
				a.m.–p.m.
				a.m.–p.m.

Charge nurse: _____

Exercise 3.1

Answer the following questions.

1. Unit A has a count of 20 patients at 1 a.m. on September 1 and 30 patients at the same time on September 2. Could the counts have been different if unit A had taken a census at 12:01 a.m. on both days?

2. Would you accept the different PCUs in the hospital taking censuses at different times as long as each unit is consistent within itself?

3. A patient transferred at 5 p.m. to unit A from unit B is counted in unit A's 12:01 a.m. census as one additional patient present. Would that patient still be included in unit B's 12:01 a.m. census?

Daily Inpatient Census

The **daily inpatient census** includes the number of inpatients present at the census-taking time each day *and* any inpatients who were both admitted after the previous census-taking time and discharged before the next census-taking time. Thus, a patient admitted to the hospital at 8 a.m. on June 1 and discharged at 10 p.m. that same day would not be present for the midnight head count. Therefore, he or she would not appear on the census report. However, the patient must be accounted for separately in some manner. For example, 20 patients are on a particular PCU. One patient was admitted at 10:00 a.m. and discharged at 7:00 p.m. If there are no other discharges, the daily inpatient census for this day is 21. You add the patient who was admitted and discharged to the 20 patients already on the unit.

Exercise 3.2

Answer the following questions.

1. The census at 12:01 a.m. on June 1 is 107. Two patients are admitted on June 1 at 6:00 a.m. and discharged at 7:00 p.m. that same day. One patient admitted at 3:00 p.m. died at 5:30 p.m. the same afternoon. What is the PCU's daily census for June 1?

2. Which would be the better form of data to keep permanently, census or daily inpatient census? Why?

3. Community Hospital's census at 12:01 a.m. on September 16 was 256. On that day, 18 patients were admitted and 22 patients were discharged. Calculate the census for September 16.

4. Community Hospital's ICU census at 12:01 a.m. on December 2 was 19. Four patients were admitted to the ICU on December 2, one was discharged to the medicine unit, and two patients died. Calculate the census for the ICU for December 2.

Inpatient Service Days

An **inpatient service day** is a unit of measure denoting the services received by one inpatient in one 24-hour period. The 24-hour period is the time between the census-taking hours on two successive days. The usual 24-hour reporting period begins at 12:01 a.m. and ends at midnight. One inpatient service day is counted for each **inpatient admission** when a patient is admitted and discharged on the same day. If this is not done, credit for the services given to that patient is lost.

There are a number of important issues concerning inpatient service days. These include:

- One unit of one service day is not usually divided or reported as a fraction of a day.

- The day of admission is counted as an inpatient service day, but the day of discharge is not.

- The days a patient does not occupy a bed due to leave of absence are excluded because he or she is not present at the census-taking hour. A **leave of absence** day is a day occurring after the admission and prior to the discharge of a hospital inpatient when the patient is not present at the census-taking hour because he or she is on leave of absence from the healthcare facility. An absence of less than one day is not considered a leave of absence in compiling statistics. A leave of absence is not common in short-term acute care hospitals because lengths of stay are usually short. However, long-term care facilities such as nursing homes, mental health facilities, drug and alcohol abuse and rehabilitation facilities, or facilities for the developmentally disabled may still use them for special reasons such as a special holiday or outing for the patient or a group of patients, a family wedding, a funeral, or if the physician is trying to determine how well a patient would fare outside the facility. Leave of absence days are always written as a physician order. When the patient or the physician believes the advantages of an absence from the facility outweigh the advantages of uninterrupted **hospitalization,** the hospital has the choice of discharging and then readmitting the patient or granting a leave of absence.

*Inpatient service d*ay is the correct term to use for what is commonly referred to as a **patient day,** inpatient day, bed occupancy day, or **census day.** The operative word here is service, that is, the number of patients who received service on a particular day. The correct wording reflects the hospital function of providing services to patients each day. If 20 patients are provided services in one 24-hour period, the number of inpatient service days for that calendar day is 20.

Exercise 3.3

Compare the definition of inpatient service day to the definitions of daily inpatient census and inpatient census. Will the figure representing an inpatient service day for any one day be the same as a daily inpatient census or inpatient census?

Total Inpatient Service Days

The term **total inpatient service days** refers to the sum of all the inpatient service days in a period under consideration. For example, if the inpatient service days for June 1, 2, and 3 are 100, 105, and 101, the total for the three days is 306. Typically, total inpatient service days are calculated monthly, quarterly, semiannually, or annually.

Exercise 3.4

Given the following inpatient service days for a 65-bed hospital, what is the total number of inpatient service days provided in June?

Date June	Inpatient Service Days	Date June	Inpatient Service Days	Date June	Inpatient Service Days
1	62	11	58	21	63
2	62	12	57	22	59
3	63	13	55	23	52
4	61	14	52	24	56
5	59	15	51	25	54
6	58	16	49	26	58
7	60	17	54	27	53
8	61	18	56	28	54
9	64	19	58	29	59
10	59	20	59	30	63

Exercise 3.5

Complete the following exercises.

1. The difference between the census and the daily inpatient census is that any patients admitted and discharged the same day are added to:

   a. The census to compute the daily inpatient census
   b. The 12:01 a.m. (or other designated time) head count to compute the daily census
   c. Both a and b
   d. None of the above

Exercise 3.5 (continued)

2. Which of the following should be used when calculating the number of inpatients who received service on a particular day?

   a. The inpatient census
   b. The daily inpatient census
   c. Total inpatient service days
   d. None of the above

3. The time for taking the inpatient census must always be:

   a. Variable
   b. Consistent
   c. 12:00 p.m.
   d. 11:59 a.m.

4. At census-taking time, a patient who has been transferred into a unit is:

   a. Counted where he or she is
   b. Counted where he or she came from
   c. Not counted
   d. Counted in both units

5. Patient day or inpatient day is more correctly termed:

   a. Inpatient service day
   b. Daily inpatient census
   c. Total inpatient service day(s)
   d. Census

6. The inpatient census at 12:01 a.m. is 57. Two patients were admitted at 1 p.m., one died at 3:15 p.m. and the other was discharged at 10:00 p.m. The inpatient service days for that day are:

   a. 50
   b. 55
   c. 57
   d. 59

7. Define the following terms:

   a. Inpatient census
   b. Daily inpatient census
   c. Inpatient service day
   d. Total inpatient service days

Calculation of Inpatient Service Days

The **calculation of inpatient service days** is the measurement of services received by all inpatients in one 24-hour period (the time between the census-taking hours on two successive days). The usual reporting period begins at 12:01 a.m. and ends at 12:00 a.m.

(midnight). Moreover, one inpatient day must be counted for each inpatient admitted and discharged on the same day between two successive census-taking hours.

> **Example:** The definitions of census, inpatient service day, and total inpatient service days provide clues for actual computation. The sample shown in table 3.2 includes all of a hospital's inpatient care units. A summary of all such units helps the administration review the hospital's overall level of activity.

> **Handy Tip:** Sometimes you may be asked by the administration to exclude PCUs such as ICUs and obstetrical units from the inpatient service days. Units such as these are studied separately because the intensity of service on these units varies greatly from the intensity of services provided on medical/surgical units. Moreover, hospital administration may want information regarding usage on these units in order to determine equipment and staffing needs. Hospitals may use inpatient service days to track trends from month to month or year-to-date.

Table 3.3 shows a sample of how hospital administration can use inpatient service days data to determine performance.

Table 3.2.   Sample inpatient service days display

Sample Inpatient Service Days	
Number of patients in hospital at 12:01 a.m. on November 1	467
Plus the number of patients admitted on November 1	+ 54
Subtotal	521
Minus the number of patients discharged (including deaths) on November 1	− 45
Number of patients in hospital at 11:59 p.m. on November 1 (subtotal)	476
Plus the number of patients both admitted and discharged on November 1	+ 3
Total inpatient service days for November 1	479

Table 3.3.   Year-to-date inpatient service days

Community Medical Center September 20XX Year-to-Date Inpatient Service Days			
Service	**Actual**	**Budget**	**Prior Year**
Medicine	12,652	15,000	14,097
Surgery	9,853	13,500	12,440
Intensive Care	2,652	3,500	2,750
Step-down	987	1,500	1,300
Rehabilitation	1,522	2,500	2,000
Obstetrics	1,621	2,200	2,160
Psychiatry	988	1,000	1,204
Newborn	1,356	1,800	1,458
Neonatal ICU	2,965	3,900	2,812
Pediatrics	528	1,000	1,523
Total	**35,124**	**45,900**	**41,744**

This medical center's analysis of its inpatient service days can be examined to determine how well the facility is doing year-to-date and compare its performance to the previous year. This can lead to discussions by administration concerning marketing of their services or examination of whether there are enough practitioners in those services that may not be doing as well as in the previous year.

Before beginning the actual calculation of census data and inpatient service days, it is important to understand the term **calculation of transfers**. The calculation of transfers occurs on the PCU census. Transfers in and out of the unit are shown as subdivisions of patients admitted to and discharged from the unit.

Example: Following are some sample figures listed in a format frequently used by the central collection area: A head count at 12:01 a.m. on June 1 shows 48 adult and children inpatients and two newborns. Using this starting point, add the number of admissions (2) and transfers in (1) to the number of adult and children inpatients (48) to arrive at a total of 51.

Note: Below, A/D indicates admitted and discharged the same day; adm, admissions; bir, births; dis, discharges; inpt, inpatients; NB, newborns; A/C, adults and children; serv, service; and trf, transfer.

| | ↓ | | + | + | ↓ | | | | | | | | | |
| | 12:01 a.m. Census | | Adm | | Trf | Total | | Dis | Dis | Trf | 11:59 p.m. Census | | | Serv Days | |
Day	A/C	NB	A/C	Bir	in	A/C	NB	A/C	NB	out	A/C	NB	A/D	A/C	NB
6/1	**48**	2	**2**	1	**1**	**51**	3	1	2	1	49	1	1	50	1

Add the births (1) to the newborns present at 12:01 a.m. to arrive at a total of three.

| | ↓ | | + | | | ↓ | | | | | | | | | |
| | 12:01 a.m. Census | | Adm | | Trf | Total | | Dis | Dis | Trf | 11:59 p.m. Census | | | Serv Days | |
Day	A/C	NB	A/C	Bir	in	A/C	NB	A/C	NB	out	A/C	NB	A/D	A/C	NB
6/1	48	**2**	2	**1**	1	51	**3**	1	2	1	49	1	1	50	1

Subtract the discharges A/C (1) and the transfers out A/C (1) from the number of adults and children (51) for an 11:59 p.m. census of 49.

| | | | | ↓ | − | − | ↓ | | | | | | | | |
| | 12:01 a.m. Census | | Adm | | Trf | Total | | Dis | Dis | Trf | 11:59 p.m. Census | | | Serv Days | |
Day	A/C	NB	A/C	Bir	in	A/C	NB	A/C	NB	out	A/C	NB	A/D	A/C	NB
6/1	48	2	2	1	1	**51**	3	**1**	2	**1**	**49**	1	1	50	1

Finally, subtract the newborns that were discharged (2) from the total number of newborns (3) for an 11:59 p.m. census of 1.

| | | | | ↓ | − | | ↓ | | | | | | | | |
| | 12:01 a.m. Census | | Adm | | Trf | Total | | Dis | Dis | Trf | 11:59 p.m. Census | | | Serv Days | |
Day	A/C	NB	A/C	Bir	in	A/C	NB	A/C	NB	out	A/C	NB	A/D	A/C	NB
6/1	48	2	2	1	1	51	**3**	1	**2**	1	49	**1**	1	50	1

The last two columns are discussed later in this chapter.

The following points should resolve any confusion:

- The terms *transfers in* and *transfers out* refer to intrahospital transfers, that is, transfers within the hospital. Transfers in and out of the hospital (called interhospital or interfacility transfers) are included in admissions and discharges. It is common for healthcare providers to use the term *transfer,* as in "The patient was transferred to the nursing home." However, this is really a discharge from the hospital and an admission to the nursing home.

- Transfers in and out of any specific medical care unit may or may not be equal, but they must be equal for the overall hospital **recapitulation.** Every patient transferred into a unit on any given day has to have been transferred out of another unit. Failure of these data to balance may mean that a unit neglected to report transfers correctly. It is essential that someone in the central collection area identify the source of error.

- The data of 49 adults and children and one newborn (the inpatient census at 11:59 p.m. on June 1) must be the same as the actual head count. If they are not the same, a unit may have reported admissions, discharges, or births incorrectly. Again, someone in the central collection area is responsible for finding the error.

- Newborns are considered separately for all computations based on census data. They should be reported separately unless otherwise directed by administration, medical staff, or other persons using the statistical data produced. Births are considered newborn admissions. As mentioned earlier, services provided to newborns differ in intensity from those provided to the rest of the hospital inpatients.

- The census at the close of one day (11:59 p.m.) is the inpatient census at the beginning of the next day and is commonly referred to as the number of patients remaining. This may be a good time to discuss the terminology used in inpatient settings. The hospital may be referred to as the "house," as in "How many patients are in the house?" This refers to the number of patients in the hospital.

Patients Admitted and Discharged on the Same Day

Going back to the last two columns from the previous problem, the number of patients who were admitted and discharged on the same day (A/D) must be added to the 11:59 p.m. census to show that they received services. These are the inpatient service days. As discussed previously, patients who are not present at either of two successive head-counting times still must be accounted for and credited with a day's care. (A patient admitted and discharged on the same day may be referred to as in and out [I&O] or admission/discharge [A&D] or any number of other terms or abbreviations.)

To compute inpatient service days, add the number of patients admitted and discharged on the same day (A/D) to the 11:59 p.m. census data. Note the 50 and 1 in the last two columns for June 1.

Handy Tip: The census for the next day must begin with the 11:59 p.m. census data and not inpatient service days. Calculate under the assumption that the patients admitted and discharged on the same day and the transfers are not newborns.

Recapitulation of Census Data

The process of verifying the data obtained by the process described previously is called the monthly or yearly recapitulation of census data, meaning a summary of the data. The total number of patients admitted and born during the month or year is added to the patients-remaining census with which the month or year began. From this sum, the number of discharges (including deaths) during the month or year is subtracted. The resulting data are the number of patients remaining at the end of the month or year. This number should equal the actual head count at 11:59 p.m. the last night of that month or year. Table 3.4 shows a sample monthly census recapitulation.

When you recap (or summarize) monthly (or annual) census data, you are verifying that the columns have been added correctly. This procedure also verifies that no error was made in the original data on one or more lines. This is accomplished by taking the 12:01 a.m. inpatient census at the beginning of the period, adding total admissions and transfers in, and subtracting total discharges and transfers out. The resultant data represent the ending census on the last day of the period (month or year).

Table 3.4.   Sample monthly census recapitulation

Community Hospital	Adults and Children	Newborns
Number of patients in hospital at 12:01 a.m. on October 1	48	2
Add the number of patients admitted in October	+ 100	+ 7
Subtotal	148	9
Subtract the number of patients discharged (including deaths) in October	− 110	− 5
Number of patients in hospital at 11:59 p.m., October 31	38	4

Exercise 3.6

Complete the following exercises.

1. Using the data given on page 31, calculate the census for June 2. Then fill in the blanks in the table below. Did the transfers in and transfers out balance?

	12:01 a.m. Census		Adm		Trf	Total		Dis	Dis	Trf	11:59 p.m. Census			Serv Days	
Day	A/C	NB	A/C	Bir	in	A/C	NB	A/C	NB	out	A/C	NB	A/D	A/C	NB
6/1	48	2	2	1	1	51	3	1	2	1	49	1			
6/2			3	1	2			4	1	2					

(continued on next page)

Exercise 3.6 (continued)

2. What data will you use to begin June 3, and why?

3. Fill in the blanks in the table below. What are the inpatient service days for June 2 and 3?

Day	12:01 a.m. Census		Adm		Trf	Total		Dis	Dis	Trf	11:59 p.m. Census		A/D	Serv Days	
	A/C	NB	A/C	Bir	in	A/C	NB	A/C	NB	out	A/C	NB		A/C	NB
6/1	48	2	2	1	1	51	3	1	2	1	49	1	1	50	1
6/2	49	1	3	1	2	54	2	4	1	2	48	1	1		
6/3			1	1	1			3	0	1			0		

4. Would a newborn ever be considered an A/D?

5. At this point, you have inpatient service days for three successive days. The total of these data, excluding newborns, for June 1, 2, and 3 is 145 (50 + 49 + 46). What will you need to know and do to get the hospital total inpatient service days for the entire month of June?

Exercise 3.7

Using the information supplied for June 1, fill in the blanks in the table below.

Day	12:01 a.m. Census		Adm		Trf	Total		Dis	Dis	Trf	11:59 p.m. Census		A/D	Serv Days	
	A/C	NB	A/C	Bir	in	A/C	NB	A/C	NB	out	A/C	NB		A/C	NB
6/1	250	18	20	4	2			25	3	2			1		
6/2			22	6	1			24	5	1			0		
6/3			24	5	0			23	4	0			3		
6/4			22	3	1			22	3	1			1		
6/5			25	4	2			25	3	2			2		

Exercise 3.8

Two hundred adults and children were in the hospital at 12:01 a.m. on August 1. There were 42 newborns at 12:01 a.m. on August 1. During August, the following data are compiled:

Admissions:

Adults and children	1,567
Newborns	97

Discharges (including deaths):

Adults and children	1,572
Newborns	107

1. What would the inpatient census for adults and children be on August 31 at 11:59 p.m.?

2. What would the inpatient census be for newborns on August 31?

3. Can the inpatient service days be computed with the information supplied in the previous question? Explain why or why not.

4. The surgery unit in Community Hospital has reported the following data. Do these data look correct? Explain.

Day	12:01 a.m. Census	Adm	Trf in	Total	Dis	Trf out	11:59 p.m. Census	A/D	Serv Days
6/1	50	6	3	59	9	1	49	1	50

Exercise 3.9

This exercise consists of two worksheets for calculating a month's inpatient census and inpatient service days. Using the data provided for May 1, complete the first worksheet. If your findings do not match the data for May 31, you have made an error either in your column additions or on one or more of the horizontal lines above the total. You must correct this error to ensure the validity of the monthly totals. If the column additions are correct, continue on to the second worksheet for the recap. This exercise could be placed on an electronic spreadsheet.

Worksheet No. 1

Day	12:01 a.m. Census A/C	NB	Adm A/C	Bir	Trf in	Total A/C	NB	Dis A/C	NB	Trf out	11:59 p.m. Census A/C	NB	A/D	Serv Days A/C	NB
1	162	2	22	1	10	194	3	19	0	10	165	3	1	166	3
2	165	3	29	0	8			23	1	8			0		
3			14	2	3			24	0	3			1		
4			24	0	5			25	0	5			0		
5			11	1	6			25	2	6			0		
6			20	0	1			16	0	1			0		
7			29	0	10			17	0	10			0		
8			24	2	13			20	0	13			3		
9			23	1	7			22	1	7			1		
10			19	0	10			17	0	10			0		
11			11	0	5			22	3	5			1		
12			16	0	6			24	0	6			0		
13			18	1	5			25	0	5			0		
14			29	0	5			19	0	5			0		
15			28	0	8			22	2	8			1		
16			26	3	6			19	0	6			0		
17			26	0	7			19	2	7			0		
18			18	0	10			25	0	10			0		
19			12	0	6			33	0	6			0		
20			22	1	8			16	3	8			1		
21			26	0	3			17	0	3			1		
22			32	2	11			25	0	11			1		
23			29	2	14			27	0	14			0		
24			22	0	10			21	2	10			0		
25			20	3	13			34	0	13			0		

Exercise 3.9 (continued)

26			14	0	6			37	1	6			1		
27			23	0	5			16	0	5			0		
28			26	2	4			18	2	4			0		
29			17	0	6			22	1	6			1		
30			19	0	7			21	1	7			0		
31			21	1	12			16	0	12	146	3	1	147	3

Worksheet No. 2

Recap of Monthly Data for Adults and Children: May 20XX
(enter numbers from Worksheet No. 1)

12:01 a.m. Census A/C		162
Adm A/C	+	_____
Trf in	+	_____
Total A/C	=	_____
Dis A/C	−	_____
Trf out	−	_____
11:59 p.m. Census A/C	=	146

Recap of Monthly Data for Newborns:

12:01 a.m. Census NB		2
Bir	+	_____
Total NB	=	_____
Dis NB	−	_____
11:59 p.m. Census NB	=	3

Serv Days A/C (total inpatient service days excluding newborns) _____

Serv Days NB (total newborn service days) _____

Total inpatient service days _____

Average Daily Inpatient Census

The **average daily inpatient census** is the average number of inpatients present each day for a given period of time. The total inpatient service days for any period (usually a month or a year) represents the inpatient service days for all the calendar days in that period. The formula for calculating average daily inpatient census is:

$$\frac{\text{Total inpatient service days for a period (excluding newborns)}}{\text{Total number of days in the period}}$$

When calculating the average daily inpatient census for a month, you need to know how many days there are in each month. Remember the nursery rhyme?

Thirty days hath September, April, June, and November.
All the rest have thirty-one.
Excepting February alone,
Which has twenty-eight days clear,
But twenty-nine each Leap Year.

Example: In the second worksheet in exercise 3.9 starting on page 37, the answer was 4,868 inpatient service days for adults and children and 91 inpatient service days for newborns for the month of May. According to the formula, the average daily inpatient census is computed by dividing 4,868 by 31 (number of days in May). The result is 157.03, or, rounded to a whole number, 157.

Handy Tip: Because patient load can fluctuate, the administration is very interested in the hospital's average daily inpatient census. For example, many healthcare facilities in southern states experience a rise in average daily inpatient census during the winter months and a decrease during the summer months due to seasonal visitors. The average daily inpatient census is a measure of use and a reference for anticipated revenues.

As mentioned earlier, adults and children are calculated separately from newborns unless otherwise directed by the hospital's administration. Newborn census data can distort statistics related to resource use. For example, it costs less to maintain a newborn nursery than it does to staff other PCUs. If the average daily inpatient census is consistently low over a specified period, it may be appropriate to close PCUs to reduce expenses. In this example, the average daily newborn census is calculated by dividing 91 by 31. The result is 2.94 or 3.

Handy Tip: Whether or not to round to a whole number is the individual hospital's decision. What is important is that the hospital act consistently. There is a difference between working with data representing people (because you cannot have a portion of a person) and working with percentages that represent numbers. Many facilities use a whole number when calculating the census and fractions with other healthcare statistics. (See chapter 2 for a discussion of rounding.)

Example: A 100-bed hospital reports 2,579 inpatient service days for October. To compute the average daily inpatient census for October, divide 2,579 by 31 (number of days in October). The average daily inpatient census is 83.19 or when rounded to a whole number is 83. This simply means that on average, 83 patients were in the facility during each day in October.

Again, this number is very important to administration because they will want to know how many patients are being served each month in order to determine staffing and supply needs for practitioners and to monitor the overall financial performance of the facility.

Average Daily Newborn Census

The formula for calculating the average daily newborn census follows the same pattern as the formula for calculating the average daily inpatient census of adults and children.

$$\frac{\textit{Total newborn inpatient service days for a period}}{\textit{Total number of days in the period}}$$

Example: A hospital with 25 bassinets had 652 newborn inpatient service days during September. Divide the total number of newborn inpatient service days (652) by the number of days in the period (30 days in September) to obtain the average daily newborn census (21.7333, or 22).

Handy Tip: When administrators and physicians ask for the average daily inpatient census, they may not always indicate to exclude newborns. Clarify the information by asking if newborns should be included or excluded from your computations.

Average Daily Inpatient Census for a Patient Care Unit

The hospital's administration often finds it helpful to know the average use of a specific medical care unit (for example, to know whether additional beds are needed for the ICU). Statistics are the basis for decision making. The formula for calculating the average daily inpatient census for a care unit is:

$$\frac{\textit{Total inpatient service days for the unit for the period}}{\textit{Total number of days in the period}}$$

Example: A hospital with a 15-bed cardiac care unit reports 450 inpatient service days for July. To compute the average daily inpatient census, divide 450 by 31 (number of days in July). The average daily inpatient census is 14.5 or 15. This indicates that the cardiac care unit is, on average, filled to capacity each day. Administration may want to consider this information closely to determine if additional beds may be needed.

Handy Tip: Some of the exercises in this textbook cover leap years. A leap year is a year in which an extra day is added to the calendar in order to harmonize with the seasons. It takes the Earth 365.2422 days to complete its course around the Sun; thus, a leap year must be added roughly once every four years. The extra day in a leap year is called a leap day and is added to the end of February, giving February 29 days. Therefore, regular years have 365 days; leap years have 366 when February 29th is added.

Exercise 3.10

Complete the following exercises.

1. Community Hospital has 200 beds and 25 newborn bassinets. The total inpatient service days for February, in a non-leap year, were 4,879 for adults and children and 658 for newborns.

    a. What is the average daily inpatient census, excluding newborns? Round to a whole number.
    b. Determine the average daily newborn census. Round to a whole number.

2. A 150-bed, 15-bassinet hospital has 3,264 inpatient service days for adults and children and 365 newborn service days during November.

    a. What is the average daily inpatient census, excluding newborns? Round to a whole number.
    b. Determine the average daily newborn census. Round to a whole number.

3. Compute the average daily newborn census for a 100-bed, 10-bassinet hospital with 2,589 inpatient service days for adults and children and 257 inpatient service days for newborns during September. Round your answer to a whole number.

4. If you need to calculate the average daily inpatient census of the surgical unit, where can you obtain the surgical unit's inpatient service days?

5. Community Hospital's burn unit has seven beds. The inpatient service days for January were 199. What is the average daily inpatient census for the burn unit during January? Round your answer to a whole number.

6. Community Hospital reports the following (round answers to whole numbers):

Community Hospital
December 20XX

	Adults and Children	Nursery
Beginning census on December 1	86	8
Admissions	248	62
Discharges and deaths	217	59
Inpatient service days	2,022	248

    a. Calculate the average daily inpatient census for adults and children.
    b. Calculate the average daily inpatient census for the nursery.
    c. What will the census for adults and children be at 11:59 p.m. on December 31?
    d. What will the newborn census be at 11:59 p.m. on December 31?

Exercise 3.10 (continued)

7. Metropolitan Hospital has a large, very busy patient care unit devoted to patients with infectious diseases. The 30-bed unit calculated the following inpatient service days for the week of February 2nd.

   Using the information below, what is the average daily inpatient census for the week of February 2 through February 8, 20XX? Round to three digits after the decimal.

**Metropolitan Hospital
Infectious Diseases Unit
Inpatient Service Days
February 2–February 8, 20XX**

Day	Inpatient Service Days
February 2	27
February 3	26
February 4	23
February 5	23
February 6	25
February 7	25
February 8	22

Chapter 3 Test

1. Differentiate between the terms *inpatient census* and *daily inpatient census*.

2. What is an intrahospital transfer?

3. Is it possible that the transfers into a patient care unit may not equal the transfers out of the same patient care unit on the same day?

4. When must transfers in and transfers out be equal?

5. At 11:59 p.m. on January 1, the Community Hospital census was 321. On January 2, 73 patients were admitted, 24 were discharged, and 3 were admitted and died that day. In their ICU unit the census on January 1 was 12. On January 2, 4 patients were admitted, 3 were discharged, and 1 was admitted and later that day died in the ICU. Answer the following questions and round the answers to whole numbers.

   a. Calculate the inpatient census for January 2.
   b. Calculate the hospital daily inpatient census for January 2.
   c. Calculate the ICU inpatient service days for January 2.

(continued on next page)

Chapter 3 Test (continued)

6. In 20XX, a hospital had 150 beds for adults and children from January 1 through June 30. On July 1, the hospital increased its beds to 200 and the number remained at 200 through December 31. During the first six months, 27,813 patient days of service were provided to the hospital's adults and children. During the last six months, 35,873 days of service were provided. Answer the following questions and round the answers to whole numbers. This is a non-leap year.

   a. What was the average daily inpatient census for the first six months: 153, 154, 155, or 156?

   b. What was the average daily inpatient census for the entire year: 173, 174, 175, or 193?

   c. The same hospital provided 7,890 newborn days of service in its 30-bassinet nursery during the year. What was the average daily newborn census: 20, 21, 22, or 23?

   d. The same hospital's surgery unit has 45 beds. During July, the unit provided 2,002 days of service. What was the average daily inpatient census for the surgery unit in July: 60, 62, 63, or 65?

7. Using the statistics from the following monthly report from the nursing administration of Community Hospital, an acute care facility, calculate the current month's (June) average daily inpatient census for each nursing unit and the totals. Note that this facility's policy is to round to a whole number.

Community Hospital
Inpatient Statistical Report
Average Daily Inpatient Census by Nursing Unit
June 20XX

	Unit	Inpatient Service Days	Average Daily Inpatient Census
A	Obstetrical	520	
B	Pediatric	87	
C	Medicine/Surgery	6,176	
D	Medicine ICU	383	
E	Surgery ICU	307	
F	Psychiatry	603	
G	Rehabilitation	725	
H	Cardiac Care Unit	213	
Total Adult and Children		**9,014**	
I	Newborn Nursery	475	
J	Special Care Nursery	135	
K	Neonatal ICU	408	
Total Nursery		**1,018**	

Chapter 4
Percentage of Occupancy

Key Terms

Bed count

Bed count day

Bed occupancy ratio

Bed turnover rate

Certificate of need

Hospital inpatient beds

Hospital newborn bassinet

Inpatient bed count

Newborn bassinet count

Observation patient

Occupancy percent

Occupancy ratio

Percent of occupancy

Percentage of occupancy

Total bed count days

Objectives

At the conclusion of this chapter, you should be able to:

- Define and differentiate among the terms inpatient bed count, bed complement, total bed count days, newborn bassinet count, bed count days, newborn bassinet count days

- Identify the beds that are included in a bed count

- Compute the bed occupancy percentage for any period given the data representing bed count and inpatient service days (adults and children)

- Compute the bassinet occupancy percentage for any period given bassinet count and newborn inpatient service days (newborn)

- Compute the percentage of occupancy for a period when there has been a change in the number of beds during that period

- Calculate the direct and indirect bed turnover rate

Inpatient Bed Count

Typically, a healthcare facility is licensed by the state to operate with a specific number of beds. When a new facility wants to open its doors for patient care, or when an existing hospital wants to add services or major medical equipment, it may need to apply to the state for a **certificate of need** (CON) to prove that patient care beds are needed in the area. Certificate of need programs are designed to contain healthcare facility costs and prevent the duplication of services and construction. Thirty-six states, the District of Columbia, and Puerto Rico require a CON program. Even the fourteen states that do not require a certificate of need have some mechanisms to regulate costs and duplication of services. When granted a CON, the facility is licensed for the specific number of beds requested and is responsible for reporting its bed count.

A **bed count,** also called an **inpatient bed count,** is the number of available **hospital inpatient beds,** both occupied and vacant, on any given day. In a hospital, the bed count includes those beds set up for normal use, whether or not they are occupied. A bed count may be reported for the entire hospital or for any of its units. Normally, when counting inpatient beds, only those in areas designed for such accommodations and set up, staffed, equipped, and in all respects ready for the care of inpatients are counted. This is an important consideration because regulatory agency surveyors often verify bed count and location against licensed beds and appropriate staffing levels. The bed count may be used in various reports, from those prepared for accrediting agencies to those prepared for regulatory agencies. In a hospital, the number of available beds in the facility or a unit may remain constant for long periods of time. At times, however, the number can change. For example, a significant number of beds may be unavailable for use during a major remodeling or renovation project, but the number will increase after the project is completed. Another example occurs during a disaster, natural or otherwise. Regular beds may be occupied, so additional beds would be set up in alcoves or hallways or other areas that are not considered patient rooms. These beds do not become a part of the regular bed count. Some facilities refer to these as disaster beds. Therefore, it is important to do a bed count.

Bed complement is an alternate term for bed count, and bed capacity sometimes is used synonymously with bed count and bed complement (although its use has led to some confusion). Bed capacity also can denote the number of beds that a facility has been designed and constructed to contain, rather than the actual number of beds set up and staffed for use. To avoid confusion, it is preferable to use bed count.

Certain types of beds excluded from the bed count are those in treatment areas such as examining rooms, emergency services, physical therapy, labor rooms, and recovery rooms.

Labor Room Beds and Newborn Beds

An obstetrics patient may be admitted directly to a labor room bed instead of to a postpartum bed where she may spend the majority of her hospital stay. Labor room beds are not included in the bed count because they are used only temporarily before the patient delivers.

Newborn beds called bassinets are computed separately from the bed count. The **newborn bassinet count** is the number of available **hospital newborn bassinets,** both occupied and vacant, on any given day.

Emergency Services Department Beds

Emergency services department (ESD) beds are normally considered outpatient beds. In some instances, however, the hospital provides an observation bed in the ESD. If observation beds meet the qualifications of being set up, equipped, and staffed for inpatient use, they may be counted in the bed count depending on what the particular facility has decided and on state-licensing compliance.

A patient under observation, an **observation patient,** needs to be monitored, evaluated, and assessed for admission to inpatient status or discharged for care to another setting. A patient can occupy a special bed set aside for this purpose or a bed in any unit of the hospital (that is, the ESD, a medical unit, or obstetrics). Usually hospital administration decides on the terms to describe and classify outpatients who occupy hospital beds and information systems to track these patients.

Exercise 4.1

In the event of a disaster, extra beds may be set up to meet the immediate needs of the situation. Would these beds be part of the bed count?

Bed Count Days

A **bed count day** is a unit of measure denoting the presence of one inpatient bed (either occupied or vacant) set up and staffed for use in one 24-hour period. The term **total bed count days** refers to the sum of inpatient bed count days for each of the days in the period under consideration. Bed count days also may be referred to as the maximum number of patient days or potential days because they represent a statistical probability of every bed being occupied every day.

> **Example:** A hospital has an inpatient bed count of 100. During September, the bed count days would be 100 (number of beds) × 30 (the number of days in September) or 3,000.

> If every hospital bed were filled each day for a certain period (for example, a month), the inpatient bed occupancy rate would be 100 percent for that month. This is because each bed was occupied the maximum number of times it could have been occupied.

We can also use this for newborn bassinets. An inpatient bassinet count day is a unit of measure denoting the presence of one inpatient bassinet (either occupied or vacant) set up and staffed for use in one 24-hour period. The term total bassinet count days refers to the sum of inpatient bassinet count days for each of the days in the period under consideration.

> **Example:** A hospital has a bassinet count of 10. The bed count days in September would be 10 (number of bassinets) × 30 (the number of days in September) or 300.

All the rates in this text can be determined by remembering this general rule: A rate is the number of times something has happened compared to the number of times something could have happened. The equation is:

$$Rate = \frac{Part}{Base}$$

or:

$$\frac{\textit{The number of times something happened}}{\textit{The number of times it could have happened}}$$

The number of times "something happened" is expressed in terms of inpatient service days. The number of times "it could have happened" is expressed in terms of bed count days (bed count multiplied by the number of calendar days). (See chapter 2 for the discussion on rates.)

Bed Occupancy Ratio/Percentage

Occupancy percentages also are referred to as rates or ratios. The **bed occupancy ratio** is the proportion of beds occupied, defined as the ratio of inpatient service days to bed count days in the period under consideration. The inpatient service days are used to represent the actual occupancy (number of times something happened) and the bed count represents the possibility for occupancy (number of times it could have happened). The formula for determining bed occupancy ratio is:

$$\frac{\textit{Total inpatient service days in a period} \times 100}{\textit{Total bed count days in the period (Bed count} \times \textit{Number of days in the period)}}$$

Synonymous terms for bed occupancy ratio are **percent of occupancy,** occupancy rate, **occupancy percent, percentage of occupancy,** and **occupancy ratio.** The ratio is usually expressed as a percent and can be computed for any specified day or as a daily average in any period of time.

Example: On June 1, 170 inpatient service days were provided in a 200-bed hospital. Making the appropriate substitutions in the previously stated formula, the bed occupancy ratio for June 1 is calculated as follows:

$$\frac{(170 \times 100)}{200} = \frac{17,000}{200} = 85\%$$

The bed occupancy ratio for June 1 is 85 percent. This simply means that on June 1, 85 percent of the beds were occupied.

Handy Tip: You might prefer to compute a decimal fraction and then multiply by 100. Another option is to convert to a percentage by moving the decimal point two places to the right as:

$$\frac{170}{200} = 0.85 = 0.85 \times 100 = 85\%$$

Another example of bed occupancy ratio for the period of a month by patient care unit is shown in the following table.

Community Hospital
December 20XX

Patient Care Unit/ Bed Count	Inpatient Service Days	Percentage of Occupancy (Rounded to One Decimal Point)
Medicine/24 beds	731	$\frac{(731 \times 100)}{(24 \times 31)} = 98.25\% = 98.3\%$
Surgery/16 beds	392	$\frac{(392 \times 100)}{(16 \times 31)} = 79.0\%$
Rehabilitation/4 beds	97	$\frac{(97 \times 100)}{(4 \times 31)} = 78.2\%$
Obstetrics/6 beds	180	$\frac{(180 \times 100)}{(6 \times 31)} = 96.77\% = 96.8\%$
Total/50 beds	1,400	$\frac{(1400 \times 100)}{(50 \times 31)} = 90.3\%$

Example: The total bed occupancy ratio for December is 90.3 percent. Additionally, as the example shows, it is possible to compute the bed occupancy rate for individual patient care units (PCUs).

In another example, a hurricane hit a small coastal town on September 19, 20XX. The local hospital is licensed for 75 beds. All 75 beds were occupied; an additional 10 beds (disaster beds) were set up in the facility and occupied. The calculation for the percentage of occupancy for September 19 would be:

$$\frac{(85 \times 100)}{(75 \times 1)} = 113.3\%$$

This is an example of an instance where the percentage of occupancy is greater than 100 percent. This often happens in a disaster. It is important to note that even though 10 additional beds were set up temporarily to handle the increased patient load, only the 75 beds are used in the denominator because they are the normal number of beds available. Remember that disaster beds or other beds set up for temporary use are not counted in the bed count.

Exercise 4.2

Using the information in the table below, calculate (round to one decimal place) the percentage of occupancy for each day of the month and for the entire month.

Community Hospital
September 20XX
75 beds

Date	Inpatient Service Days	Percentage of Occupancy	Date	Inpatient Service Days	Percentage of Occupancy
1	74		16	62	
2	73		17	61	
3	70		18	78	
4	71		19	75	
5	68		20	76	
6	67		21	77	
7	66		22	79	
8	54		23	72	
9	59		24	64	
10	69		25	58	
11	49		26	65	
12	52		27	63	
13	55		28	60	
14	56		29	53	
15	57		30	51	

Exercise 4.3

Using the information in the table below, calculate (round to one decimal place) the percentage of occupancy for each unit of Children's Hospital as well as the total percentage of occupancy.

Children's Hospital
April 20XX

Unit	Bed Count	Inpatient Service Days	Percentage of Occupancy
Pediatric Medicine	55	1,450	
Pediatric Surgery	40	1,059	
Respiratory	25	642	
Hematology/Oncology	38	1,122	
Pediatric ICU	12	275	
Pediatric Cardiac ICU	10	261	
Neonatal ICU	20	456	
Total			

Change in Bed Count

Occasionally, a hospital changes its bed count during a period of time. This expansion or reduction would be considered a permanent change and is not designed to meet a temporary or emergency situation.

For example, a hospital changes its official bed count from 50 to 75 on January 15 and goes on to provide a total of 1,700 inpatient service days for the entire month. How is the maximum number of bed count days determined for the month of January? Multiply 50 beds by the first 14 days of the month and 75 beds by the remaining 17 days of the month, and then add the products.

$$14 \times 50 = 700$$
$$17 \times 75 = 1,275$$
$$700 + 1,275 = 1,975$$

The maximum number of bed count days for January is 1,975. Now compute the bed occupancy ratio. The calculation is:

$$\frac{(1,700 \times 100)}{1,975} = \frac{170,000}{1,975} = 86.07\% = 86.1\%$$

The bed occupancy ratio for January is 86.1 percent.

This procedure provides the most accurate result. Compare the previous computation with what would have happened if 50 beds had been used for the entire month. The calculation is:

$$\frac{(1,700 \times 100)}{(50 \times 31)} = \frac{170,000}{1,550} = 109.67 = 109.7\%$$

If 75 beds had been used for the entire month, the calculation would be:

$$\frac{(1,700 \times 100)}{(75 \times 31)} = \frac{170,000}{2,325} = 73.11 = 73.1\%$$

Obviously, there is a significant difference in the results. This example illustrates how easy it can be to present an inaccurate statistical picture. Because many administrative decisions are made on the basis of statistical presentations, the health information management (HIM) practitioner has an important responsibility in providing accurate data and validating computerized statistics.

Exercise 4.4

Community Hospital began the year 20XX, a non-leap year, with 102 beds. On March 1st, it had expanded the number of beds to 116. From April 1st through June 30th, the hospital reported 120 beds. The hospital increased to 124 beds from July 1st through October 31st. Finally, the hospital completed its expansion process on November 1st to end the year with 130 beds. Use these data to answer the questions below. Round to one decimal place.

Community Hospital
Annual Statistics, 20XX

Month	Bed Count (A/C)	Inpatient Service Days	Percentage of Occupancy
January	102	2,895	
February	102	2,796	
March	116	2,991	
April	120	3,078	
May	120	3,087	
June	120	3,396	
July	124	3,587	
August	124	3,656	
September	124	3,654	
October	124	3,698	
November	130	3,832	
December	130	3,765	

Exercise 4.4 (continued)

1. Calculate the percentage of occupancy for each month.

2. Calculate the percentage of occupancy for each quarter (January through March, April through June, July through September, and October through December).

3. Calculate the percentage of occupancy for the year.

Exercise 4.5

Using the statistics in the following report generated for Community Hospital, calculate (round to one decimal place) the percentage of occupancy for the month of December.

Community Hospital
December 20XX

PCU	Inpatient Service Days	Bed Count	Percentage of Occupancy
Med/Surg	1,876	70	
ICU	300	10	
CCU	240	8	
Rehabilitation	300	12	
Burn	75	5	
Psychiatry	200	15	
Pediatric	870	30	
Total			
Nursery	280	10	

Newborn Bassinet Occupancy Ratio

Typically, newborn occupancy ratios are computed separately. If every bassinet were full every day in the period, the hospital would have the maximum potential bassinet occupancy. The formula for determining newborn bassinet occupancy is:

$$\frac{Total\ newborn\ inpatient\ service\ days\ for\ a\ period \times 100}{Total\ newborn\ bassinet\ count \times Number\ of\ days\ in\ the\ period}$$

Example: During March, a hospital with a bassinet count of 30 provided 810 newborn inpatient service days of care. According to the formula, the newborn bassinet occupancy ratio for March would be:

$$\frac{(810 \times 100)}{(30 \times 31)} = \frac{81,000}{930} = 87.09\% = 87.1\%$$

Exercise 4.6

Use the statistics in the following report generated for Community Hospital to make the following three calculations (non-leap year). Round to one decimal place.

Community Hospital
Annual Statistics, 20XX

Newborn bassinets
January–March: 10
April–June: 12
July–September: 15
October–December: 20

Month	Newborn Inpatient Service Days	Percentage of Occupancy
January	300	
February	280	
March	307	
April	326	
May	355	
June	340	
July	427	
August	415	
September	430	
October	452	
November	444	
December	495	

1. Calculate the percentage of occupancy for each month.

2. Calculate the percentage of occupancy for each quarter (January through March, April through June, July through September, and October through December).

3. Calculate the percentage of occupancy for the year.

Bed Turnover Rate

The **bed turnover rate** refers to the number of times a bed, on average, changes occupants during a given period of time or the average number of admissions per bed per time period. The bed turnover rate is useful because two time periods may have the same percentage of occupancy, but the turnover rates may be different. For example, if a unit such as an obstetrics unit has a high turnover rate, this could be an indication that the unit can accommodate more patients because the patients have a shorter length of stay (LOS). Conversely, a rehabilitation unit might have a low turnover rate because the patients in that unit have a longer

LOS. The bed turnover rate is a measure of the frequency of bed use. It demonstrates the net effect of changes in occupancy rate and LOS. (See chapter 5 for a discussion of LOS.) Following are two formulas for determining bed turnover rate. The direct formula is:

$$\frac{Number\ of\ discharges\ (including\ deaths)\ for\ a\ period}{Average\ bed\ count\ during\ the\ period}$$

The indirect formula is:

$$\frac{Occupancy\ rate\ \times\ Number\ of\ days\ in\ a\ period}{Average\ length\ of\ stay}$$

Although there is no universal agreement on the most accurate formula, administrators of short-stay hospitals are becoming increasingly interested in bed turnover rate as a measure of hospital services used, especially when related as a rate to occupancy and LOS. When occupancy goes up and LOS goes down, or vice versa, the bed turnover rate makes it easier to see the net effect of these changes.

Turnover rates can be used in comparing one facility with another or in comparing utilization rates for different time periods or for different units of the same facility. For example, the occupancy rate for one hospital can be essentially the same in two time periods, but the turnover rate may be lower because of a longer LOS in one time period. In other words, bed turnover rate can be a measure of intensity of utilization.

Exercise 4.7 displays both formulas and yields basically the same turnover rate for a short-stay hospital.

Exercise 4.7

Community Hospital
Annual Statistics, 20XX
Non-leap year
200 beds

Patients discharged (includes deaths): 6,500
Average length of stay: 9 days
Bed occupancy rate: 80 percent

1. Apply the direct formula for the turnover rate. Round to one decimal place.

2. Apply the indirect formula for the turnover rate. Round to one decimal place.

Answers:

Turnover rate (direct formula):

Turnover rate (indirect formula):

Exercise 4.8

Match the description with the definition:

1. _____   CON—Certificate of Need
2. _____   Bed Count/Inpatient Bed Count
3. _____   Bed Capacity
4. _____   Bed Count Day
5. _____   Total Bed Count Days
6. _____   Bed Occupancy Ratio
7. _____   Bed Turnover Rate

A. The number of available hospital inpatient beds

B. Denotes the number of beds a facility has been designed and constructed for

C. The sum of inpatient bed count days for each of the days in a period

D. May be required when a hospital wants to add a major piece of medical equipment

E. Percent of Occupancy, Percentage of Occupancy, Occupancy Ratio

F. The number of times a bed, on average, changes occupants for a period, or the average number of admissions per bed per time period

G. A unit of measure denoting the presence of one inpatient bed set up and staffed for one 24-hour period

Chapter 4 Test

A hospital compiled the following annual statistics for 20XX (non-leap year):

**Community Hospital
Annual Statistics, 20XX**

	Inpatient Service Days	Bed Count
January–June	32,785	175
July–December	34,986	200
December 31 only	201	200
Newborn	12,372	40

Select the correct answer to each of the following questions, rounding to one decimal place.

1. The inpatient occupancy rate (without newborns) for 20XX was:

    a. 18.5%
    b. 37.4%
    c. 98.7%
    d. 99.0%

Chapter 4 Test (continued)

2. The newborn bassinet occupancy rate for 20XX was:

   a. 80.4%
   b. 84.7%
   c. 84.8%
   d. 85.2%

3. The bed occupancy rate for December 31 was:

   a. 77.1%
   b. 92.5%
   c. 100.0%
   d. 100.5%

The following table is a report of the first quarter of 20XX (January–March) from a 450-bed medical center regarding its insurance categories. Round all to one decimal place. This is a non-leap year. Use this table to answer questions 4, 5, and 6.

Community Medical Center
Inpatient Service Days and Number of Discharges
by Insurance Category
January–March 20XX

Insurance Category	Inpatient Service Days	Number of Discharges
Third-party Contracts	4,859	666
Medicare	7,249	1,204
Medicaid	12,365	1,925
County Coverage	4,320	792
Private Pay	3,465	321
No Insurance	1,589	289
Total	**33,847**	**5,197**

4. Calculate the occupancy rate for:

   a. Total
   b. Medicare
   c. Private pay

5. Using the direct formula, calculate the bed turnover rate for:

   a. Total
   b. Medicare
   c. Private pay

6. What is the total average daily inpatient census for this period of time?

(continued on next page)

Chapter 4 Test (continued)

7. The following table is a report of the annual inpatient service days of Community Hospital for 20XX. The hospital has an inpatient bed count of 210 and a bassinet count of 30. Calculate (round to one decimal place) the percentage of occupancy for each month for adults/children and for newborns. This is a non-leap year.

**Community Hospital
Annual Statistics, 20XX**

| Month | Inpatient Service Days | | Percentage of Occupancy | |
	Adult/Children	Newborn	Adult/Children	Newborn
January	4,682	752		
February	4,798	798		
March	4,626	701		
April	4,876	688		
May	4,768	724		
June	4,591	743		
July	4,423	825		
August	4,234	796		
September	4,394	802		
October	4,412	865		
November	4,691	921		
December	4,832	912		
Total				

Chapter 5
Length of Stay

Key Terms

Admission date

Average duration of hospitalization

Average length of stay

Days of stay

Discharge date

Discharge days

Duration of inpatient hospitalization

Inpatient days of stay

Leave of absence day

Length of stay

Military time

Total length of stay

Utilization management

Objectives

At the conclusion of this chapter, you should be able to:

- Define the terms length of stay and discharge days
- Compute the length of stay for one patient based on data provided
- Calculate the total length of stay for a group of discharged patients
- Compute average length of stay
- Compute the average length of stay for newborns
- Describe a leave of absence day and identify when it is used in calculations

Length of Stay

Length of stay (LOS) is the number of calendar days a patient stays in the hospital, from admission to discharge. The healthcare facility uses LOS data in utilization management. **Utilization management** is a program that evaluates the facility's efficiency in providing necessary services in the most cost-effective manner, including LOS, while also evaluating the level of care required. Its goal is to eliminate over- and underutilization of services. Part of the utilization management process involves reviewing LOS for continued medical necessity. For example, is it more appropriate to continue to treat the patient in an acute care facility or to transfer the patient to a subacute or rehabilitation facility?

LOS data also are used in financial reporting, for example, to compare patients within the same Medicare Severity Diagnosis Related Group (MS-DRG). A particular MS-DRG **average length of stay (ALOS)** can be compared to the overall healthcare facility's MS-DRG ALOS to determine whether there are too many extreme values, or outliers. LOS data for patients with the same diagnosis or procedure treated by various physicians are compared to evaluate any extremes. For example, it is important for hospital administration to be aware of physician differences in LOS because these may be indicative of different types of treatment for the same condition by different physicians.

Discharge Days

Chapter 3 introduced the concept of inpatient service days, which are compiled while the patient is hospitalized. This chapter discusses **discharge days,** which are days calculated after the patient has been discharged from the hospital. Other terms for length of stay include **days of stay, inpatient days of stay,** and **duration of inpatient hospitalization.**

A discharge occurs at the end of the patient's hospital stay. Discharges include deaths, so the term *discharge* may refer to both patients who leave the hospital alive and those who have died. Often patients are transferred to other facilities to continue their care. Hospital staff may refer to these patients as transfers but they are counted as discharges.

In general, every day that a patient is in the hospital is counted as a day except the day of discharge. The LOS for one patient is determined by subtracting the **admission date** from the **discharge date** *when the patient is admitted and discharged within the same month*. The day of admission is counted in computing the number of discharge days or LOS, but the day of discharge is not.

For longer stays when the patient's stay extends beyond one or more months, days must be added to calculate the LOS.

> **Example:** For a patient admitted on January 30 and discharged on February 4, subtract January 30 from January 31 and add the 4 days in February ($31 - 30 = 1 + 4$ days in February = 5 days). The LOS is one day if the patient is admitted and discharged on the same day. These types of patients are also called admissions and discharges (A&Ds) or in and outs.

Table 5.1 shows how to calculate the LOS for a sampling of discharged patients.

Table 5.1.   Example LOS calculation

Date Admitted	Date Discharged	Length of Stay
6/25	6/25	1 day
6/25	6/26	1 day (6/26 – 6/25 = 1 day)
6/25	6/30	5 days (6/30 – 6/25 = 5 days)
6/25	7/4	9 days (5 days in June + 4 days in July = 9 days)
6/25	8/4	40 days (5 days in June + 31 days in July + 4 days in August = 40 days)

Exercise 5.1

Calculate the LOS for the following discharged patients in an acute care facility.

Date Admitted	Date Discharged	Length of Stay
5/3	5/4	
7/2	7/12	
2/14	2/28	
3/25	4/15	
8/27	9/10	

Exercise 5.2

Calculate the LOS for the following discharged patients in this long-term care facility. Keep in mind that 2008 is a leap year.

Date Admitted	Date Discharged	Length of Stay
1/1/08	11/29/08	
4/17/07	12/01/08	
6/28/08	1/9/09	
2/1/08	4/8/09	
11/29/08	6/7/09	

It is possible to calculate LOS in an outpatient facility or physician's office. For example, a patient arrived at 8:05 a.m. and was taken to the examining room at 8:22 a.m. Because the hour is the same in both cases (8 a.m.), simply subtract the minutes (22 – 05 = 17 minutes). This patient waited 17 minutes before being taken to the examining room.

If a patient arrived at 8:05 a.m. and was taken into the examining room at 9:15 a.m., subtract the minutes first (15 – 05 = 10 minutes) and then subtract the hour (9 – 8 = 1). The patient waited 1 hour and 10 minutes. Note that the second set of minutes, the taken time (15), is greater than the first set of minutes (05), the arrived time.

If the first set of minutes (arrived) is greater than the second set of minutes (taken), additional steps must take place. Subtract one hour from the second hour (taken) and increase the number of minutes on the second time by 60. Sounds a little confusing, but the following should clear up the issue. Let's say a patient arrived at 1:11 p.m. and was taken to the examining room at 3:02 p.m. The "arrival" minutes of 11 are greater than the "taken" minutes of 02.

- Subtract one hour from 3:02 which will equal 2:02
- Now the one hour (60 minutes) you took from the 3:02 needs to be added to the :02
- The "time" is now 2:62. It is now possible to subtract the 1:11 from 2:62
- 2:62 – 1:11 = 1 hour and 51 minutes, which was the patient's wait time

The next two calculations concern the amount of time between two times when one is before 12:59 and one is after 12:59. Consider this first example: A patient arrived at the physician's office at 11:47 a.m. and was taken to the examination room at 1:27 p.m.

- First add 12 hours to the time that occurred after 12:59. In this case that would be 1:27 + 12 = 13:27. This changes the time to **military time.**
- Next, note that the "arrived" minutes (47) are greater than the "taken" minutes (27)
- Subtract one hour from the 13:27. This equals 12:27
- Add the 60 minutes from that hour to the "taken" minutes. This would be 27 + 60 = 87
- The "time" in now 12:87
- Then, subtract 11:47 from 12:87. That is 12 – 11 = 1 and 87 – 47 = 40
- The patient waited 1 hour and 40 minutes

Consider this second example: A patient arrives at the outpatient clinic at 11:21 a.m. and is taken to the examination room at 2:33 p.m.

- In this case, first add 12 hours to the time that occurred after 12:59. This would be 2:33 + 12 = 14:33
- Note that the "arrived" minutes (21) are less than the "taken" minutes of 33
- Subtract the minutes 33 – 21 = 12
- Now, subtract the 11:00 from 14:00 which equals 3
- The patient waited 3 hours and 12 minutes

Exercise 5.3

1. Calculate the time it takes to see patients in this physician's office.

Time Admitted	Time Seen by Physician	Time between Checking In at Reception and Being Seen by Physician
8:00 a.m.	8:17 a.m.	
1:22 p.m.	2:05 p.m.	
10:30 a.m.	11:43 a.m.	

2. Metropolitan Hospital, a very large urban hospital, promises patients that there will be no more than a 60-minute wait between the time they arrive (sign in) at the Emergency Services Department (ESD) until they are triaged. Calculate the wait time between arrival and triage. The hospital selected eight patients at random to check the times.

   a. Calculate the wait time for each patient.
   b. What is the average wait time?
   c. Is the hospital in compliance with its own guidelines?

Patient 02.04.2012	Time of Arrival (Time "A")	Time Patient Was Triaged (Time "B")	Wait Time
Patient A	8:00 a.m.	8:18 a.m.	
Patient B	8:30 a.m.	8:55 a.m.	
Patient C	9:26 a.m.	10:47 a.m.	
Patient D	10:02 a.m.	1:25 p.m.	
Patient E	11:45 a.m.	2:04 p.m.	
Patient F	1:15 p.m.	1:59 p.m.	
Patient G	2:30 p.m.	3:10 p.m.	
Patient H	2:45 p.m.	3:50 p.m.	

Total Length of Stay

The **total length of stay** is the sum of the days' stay of any group of inpatients discharged during a specified period of time. Total length of stay also may be referred to as total discharge days. Although the total length of stay and inpatient service days may approximate each other over a long period of time, they are not interchangeable. The reason for this is that inpatient service days are counted concurrently and discharge days are counted after discharge.

Example: A patient hospitalized for a period beyond an entire year and into a second year (for example, a rehabilitation patient) would be credited with 365 inpatient service days at the end of the first year, but no discharge days. When the patient is discharged from the hospital in the second year, all the discharge days from admission to discharge are counted at that time, increasing the discharge days for the second year by at least 365.

If the patient stays in the hospital for two or more years (as often happens in long-term facilities), all 730+ discharge days are assigned to one year in calculating the duration of inpatient hospitalization. These types of patients increase the number of discharge days for any year, making the total number much larger than inpatient service days for the same period.

Why calculate both inpatient days of service and total length of stay? Each is meaningful in its own right. Inpatient service days are useful in the analysis of current utilization of hospital facilities related to the entire hospital, a clinical unit, or a service department. They are used to compute various daily averages and occupancy ratios. The total length of stay can be used to analyze LOS for groups of discharged patients with similar characteristics such as age, disease, treatment, clinical service, or day of week admitted.

Exercise 5.4

Using the table below, calculate the LOS for each individual patient and then the total length of stay for the 15 patients listed at Community Hospital.

All patients were discharged on 9/20/20XX (non-leap year).

**Community Hospital
Discharge List
September 20, 20XX**

Pt. Name	Age	Clinical Service	Admission Date	Length of Stay
Anderson	72	Medicine	9/18	
Bretz	43	Surgery	8/19	
Clemments	32	Obstetrics	9/18	
Dimmick	25	Obstetrics	9/18	
Erichson	98	Medicine	9/1	
Frye	67	Medicine	8/12	
Grell	43	Surgery	9/2	
Hallbauer	15	Obstetrics	9/19	
Imel	33	Medicine	9/17	
Jordan	51	Medicine	9/16	
Kirkpatrick	23	Obstetrics	9/17	
Locke	57	Surgery	8/3	
Miller	48	Surgery	8/31	
Nickel	59	Medicine	9/4	
Oller	63	Medicine	9/9	
Total				

Exercise 5.4 (continued)

Finally, calculate the total length of stay for:

- Medicine service patients
- Surgery service patients
- Obstetrics service patients
- Patients 25 and younger
- Patients 26–40 years old
- Patients 41–55 years old
- Patients 56–70 years old
- Patients over age 70

Average Length of Stay

The average length of stay (ALOS) is the average number of days that inpatients discharged during the period under consideration stayed in the hospital. The formula for calculating ALOS is:

$$\frac{\textit{Total length of stay (discharge days)}}{\textit{Total discharges (including deaths)}}$$

In general, inpatient LOS is decreasing. Several trends in healthcare have contributed to this reduction in ALOS, including managed care, home care, skilled nursing units in hospitals, and an increase in outpatient visits. Synonymous terms for ALOS include **average duration of hospitalization** and average stay.

The formula above does not include the length of stay for newborns. Most hospitals calculate the ALOS for newborns separately because newborns ordinarily stay the same length of time as their mothers. In addition, when compared to many other classifications of patients, normal newborn stays are relatively short. In contrast, newborn stays in the newborn intensive care unit tend to be quite long, sometimes months at a time. Therefore, inclusion of both mothers and newborns would distort the total ALOS.

Exercise 5.5

Complete the following exercises.

1. In February, Community Hospital reported 825 discharge days for adults and children and 96 discharge days for newborns. During the month, 158 adults and children and 32 newborns were discharged. Calculate (round to one decimal place) the ALOS for adults and children for the month of February.

(continued on next page)

Exercise 5.5 (continued)

2. Using the table in exercise 5.4, compute the ALOS for the group of patients between ages 41 and 55. The ALOS is 18.5 days. True or false?

3. Using the report below from University Hospital for May 20XX, calculate (round to one decimal place) the ALOS for each service.

University Hospital
May 20XX

Clinical Units	Discharges	Discharge Days	ALOS
Surgery	1,720	8,627	
Medicine	1,594	7,852	
Neurology	988	4,285	
Oncology	878	18,588	
Obstetrics/Gynecology	588	1,479	
Ophthalmology	385	1,154	
Orthopedics	651	9,321	
Pediatrics	358	2,841	
Psychiatry	156	4,697	
Rehabilitation	321	8,057	
Urology	89	183	
Total			

Average Newborn Length of Stay

As stated earlier, newborn LOS is usually calculated separately. The formula for calculating average newborn LOS is:

$$\frac{\textit{Total newborn discharge days}}{\textit{Total newborn discharges (including deaths)}}$$

Exercise 5.6

Using the table below, calculate (round to one decimal place) the ALOS for newborns in each month and then compute the annual ALOS.

University Hospital
Annual Newborn Discharge Statistics
20XX

Month	Newborn Discharges	Discharge Days	Newborn ALOS
January	95	238	
February	120	348	
March	112	347	
April	135	540	
May	142	454	
June	137	369	
July	176	616	
August	189	429	
September	207	601	
October	198	555	
November	152	501	
December	135	405	
Total			

Leave of Absence Days

Another data element that is significant in some hospitals is the number of leave of absence days. A **leave of absence** is a physician-authorized absence of an inpatient from a hospital or other facility for a specified period of time occurring after admission and prior to discharge. This means that the physician writes an order that the patient can have a leave of absence.

A **leave of absence day** is determined when the patient is not present at the census-taking hour. A leave of absence involves an overnight pass, or, more frequently given in longer-stay facilities, a weekend pass; thus, the patient would not be present when the census is taken.

Leave of absence data are important for administrative purposes as well as for the analysis of the services provided and care patterns. Leave of absence days are usually excluded or tabulated separately when computing bed occupancy, calculating inpatient service days, or preparing an inpatient census. Another issue with leave of absence days is that insurance companies generally do not pay for days outside the hospital. Thus, if the days are being used in conjunction with financial data, they may need to be separated from the actual days in the hospital. However, they are included when considering discharge days and computing ALOS. Hospitals that generally have longer lengths of stay, such as rehabilitation, mental health, or chronic care hospitals, will use the leave of absence as a way for the patient to adjust to time away from the facility, so it is considered to be part of the patient's treatment. If the leave of absence is not considered part of the patient treatment, the physician may elect to discharge and then readmit the patient rather than grant a leave of absence.

Exercise 5.7

Using the statistics in the tables below, determine the following calculations for Community Hospital.

1. Compute the LOS for each of the patients in the table below. (Remember that 2008 was a leap year.) If no year is specified, assume it is not a leap year and both dates are in the same year.

Admitted	Discharged	LOS
1/12	1/31	
7/4	7/30	
1/1/2008	2/1/2009	
11/24	11/24	
6/19/2007	1/4/2009	

2. What is the total length of stay for this group of patients?

Using the information in the table below, answer questions 3 through 7. Round to one decimal place.

Community Hospital
Annual Statistics, 20XX

	Number of Discharges	Discharge Days
Total Adults and Children	15,987	92,725
Total Newborns	3,421	11,062
The following services are included in the above totals:		
Medicine	11,644	51,201
Surgery	4,852	32,103
Obstetrics	2,912	10,483

3. Compute the ALOS for adult and children patients.

4. Compute the ALOS for newborn patients.

5. Compute the ALOS for medicine patients.

6. Compute the ALOS for surgery patients.

7. Compute the ALOS for obstetrics patients.

Exercise 5.7 (continued)

Answers:

Adults and Children ALOS:

Newborns ALOS:

Medicine ALOS:

Surgery ALOS:

Obstetrics ALOS:

8. Calculate the ALOS for the following Medicare patients.

**Community Hospital
Medicare Discharge Statistics
July 20XX**

Unit	Medicare Discharges	Medicare Discharge Days	ALOS
Medicine	325	2,375	
Surgery	175	2,103	
Rehabilitation	298	4,179	
Skilled Nursing	305	6,588	

Chapter 5 Test

Last month, Community Hospital compiled the discharge statistics shown in the following table. Notice that the last three days are missing. Prepare a spreadsheet on a software program and enter the information from the chart. Then use the discharge lists for May 29, 30, and 31 to enter the missing data into the appropriate columns for medicine, surgery, obstetrics, and newborn discharged patients and their corresponding discharge days.

(continued on next page)

Chapter 5 Test (continued)

Finally, compute the ALOS for medicine service, surgery service, OB service, and NB service and then compute the ALOS for adults and children (medicine, surgery, and OB).

**Community Hospital
Discharge List
May 29, 20XX**

Patient Name	Age	Service	Admission Date	LOS
Andres, Michael	74	Medicine	5-20	9
Barty, Stephen	43	Surgery	5-18	11
Christenson, Andrea	27	OB	5-27	2
Christenson, Baby Boy	NB	NB	5-27	2
Denison, William	51	Surgery	5-9	20
Henry, Christopher	76	Surgery	5-15	14
Jackson, Michelle	19	OB	5-26	3
Katon, Marie	39	OB	5-27	2
Williamson, Baby Boy	NB	NB	5-24	5

**Community Hospital
Discharge List
May 30, 20XX**

Patient Name	Age	Service	Admission Date	LOS
Adams, Paul	43	Medicine	5-26	4
Butler, Thomas	56	Medicine	5-28	2
Carson, Johnnie	76	Surgery	5-25	5
Daniels, George	54	Medicine	5-27	3
George, Michael	23	Surgery	5-26	4
Hanson, Joyce	19	OB	5-28	2
Hanson, Baby Girl	NB	NB	5-28	2
Jacquinta, Marlene	20	OB	5-26	4
Jacquinta, Baby Boy	NB	NB	5-26	4
Katosh, Joseph	67	Medicine	5-27	3
Kettison, Jack	39	Medicine	5-25	5
Kettison, Mary	67	Surgery	5-27	3
Laytham, Clint	60	Surgery	5-27	3

Chapter 5 Test (continued)

Matson, Dorianne	67	Medicine	5-28	2
Nettleson, Andy	34	Surgery	5-26	4
Otto, Pierce	78	Medicine	5-27	3
Ransom, Jackson	45	Medicine	5-25	5
Springer, Mary	56	Surgery	5-28	2
Tatum, Neal	34	Surgery	5-28	2
Wallace, Mattie	29	OB	5-30	1
Zininsky, Maureen	22	OB	5-29	1

**Community Hospital
Discharge List
May 31, 20XX**

Patient Name	Age	Service	Admission Date	LOS
Allan, Randy	42	Medicine	5-26	4
Banta, Janet	43	Medicine	5-25	6
Cox, David	78	Surgery	5-29	2
Dunning, Stephen	12	Surgery	5-28	3
Epp, Melvin	56	Medicine	5-24	7
Farmer, Jaimie	23	OB	5-28	3
Farmer, Baby Girl	NB	NB	5-28	3
Finney, G. W.	55	Surgery	5-27	4
Fry, Benedict	38	Surgery	5-28	3
Girard, Katherine	37	Medicine	5-29	2
Halford, Harold	55	Surgery	5-28	3
Kilpatrick, Susan	19	OB	5-28	3
Kilpatrick, Baby Boy	NB	NB	5-28	3
Martindale, Amanda	23	OB	5-28	3
Martindale, Baby Boy	NB	NB	5-28	3
McLoughlin, Baby Boy	NB	NB	5-27	4
Nachtigall, Brian	27	Medicine	5-27	4
Niazi, Baby Boy	NB	NB	5-27	4
Poepperling, Wanda	65	Medicine	5-28	3
Trotman, Baby Girl	NB	NB	5-30	1

(continued on next page)

Chapter 5 Test (continued)

Community Hospital
Student Name
May 20XX

Date	Medicine		Surgery		Obstetrics		Subtotal		Newborn		Total	
	No. Pts.	Dis Days	No. Pts.	Dis Days	No. Pts.	Dis Days	No. Pts.	Dis Days	No. Pts.	Dis Days	No. Pts.	Dis Days
1-May	12	36	5	23	2	8			3	12		
2-May	8	40	2	25	5	16			6	23		
3-May	6	36	8	80	3	10			3	10		
4-May	4	21	4	23	1	4			1	4		
5-May	11	47	3	42	4	10			4	10		
6-May	15	77	5	23	3	7			2	5		
7-May	6	52	7	56	2	5			3	7		
8-May	5	71	9	123	6	13			5	10		
9-May	8	63	1	4	3	9			2	13		
10-May	9	72	4	26	2	6			3	9		
11-May	7	34	9	112	3	8			3	8		
12-May	2	9	3	27	1	2			1	2		
13-May	5	28	4	16	2	5			1	3		
14-May	4	29	6	119	2	7			2	7		
15-May	9	26	8	95	2	6			2	6		
16-May	7	45	4	81	4	8			5	11		
17-May	6	37	2	15	3	8			3	8		
18-May	4	52	9	37	3	10			2	10		
19-May	8	63	3	37	2	6			3	9		
20-May	3	29	5	23	1	3			0	0		
21-May	5	35	8	78	4	9			4	9		
22-May	5	34	4	32	2	4			3	8		
23-May	8	53	1	5	3	6			3	6		
24-May	7	26	2	62	2	4			2	4		
25-May	2	23	3	42	4	12			2	7		
26-May	3	23	4	53	2	5			3	9		
27-May	5	25	2	10	3	10			4	11		
28-May	9	38	6	75	1	3			2	8		
29-May												
30-May												
31-May												
Total	183	1124	131	1344	75	204			77	229		

Chapter 6
Death (Mortality) Rates

Key Terms

Anesthesia death rate

Cancer mortality rate

Case fatality rate

Centers for Medicare and Medicaid Services

Complication

Crude death rate

Dead on arrival

Death rate

Disposition

Early fetal death

Fetal death

Fetal death rate

Gross death rate

Hospital death rate

Hospital live birth

Infant death

Institutional death rate

Intermediate fetal death

Late fetal death

Maternal death

Maternal death rate

Mortality

Mortality rate

Neonatal death

Neonatal period

Net death rate

Newborn

Newborn death

Newborn death rate

Newborn mortality rate

Perinatal death

Postneonatal death

Postoperative death rate

Postpartum

Prepartum

Stillbirth

Surgical death rate

Surgical operation

Surgical procedure

World Health Organization (WHO)

Objectives

At the conclusion of this chapter, you should be able to:

- Define and calculate the following death rates: gross, net, postoperative, anesthesia, maternal, newborn, and fetal

- Calculate the case fatality rate

- Differentiate between operation and procedure

- Define cancer mortality and calculate its rate

Death Rates

The **death rate** is the proportion of inpatient discharges that end in death, usually expressed as a percentage. The **hospital death rate** is defined as the number of inpatient deaths for a given period of time divided by the total number of live discharges and deaths for the same time period. A synonymous term for hospital death rate is **gross death rate.**

Death rates have always been important information for health agencies and hospitals in evaluating the quality of medical care. Death rate information is used by a variety of industries in addition to healthcare. For example, the automobile industry uses death rate information to determine the likelihood of drivers and passengers dying in some car models compared to others. Handgun advocates look at death rates to determine the likelihood of someone dying a violent death while using a firearm. Organizations such as the American Heart Association, the American Cancer Association, and other groups are interested in looking at death rates to help bring attention to their causes. Researchers use death rates to show causes of death in certain populations. All this information can help improve the quality of medical care given to patients.

An interesting article in the *Journal of the American Medical Association* calling for more emphasis on a new medical specialty—intensive care specialists, or intensivists—showed that having such intensive care experts could reduce death rates. The study showed that having high numbers of intensivists was associated with lower hospital mortality and lower intensive care unit (ICU) mortality (Pronovost et al. 2002). The patients cared for by intensivists had reduced ICU and hospital death rates and lengths of stay (LOS). Health information management (HIM) practitioners—and anyone else who relies on statistical information—must remember that numbers count, not only in reports and records, but also in the human equation.

Death rate data also are important in helping public health agencies plan for health services. For example, the **Centers for Medicare and Medicaid Services** (CMS) publishes information on death rates among Medicare patients, specific ethnic groups, and patients in particular diagnosis categories, to name a few. Some years ago, CMS published a report for each hospital on Medicare deaths. Initially, the CMS **mortality** data received a great deal of media coverage and caused concern in facilities because of the high percentages reported. Moreover, the report created confusion about definitions and interpretation of the data. Hospitals were permitted to correct the data, and since the initial releases, the report format has been modified. This demonstrates the importance of the HIM practitioner's need to understand death rates. HIM practitioners must understand basic death rates and be ready to calculate or verify other data pertaining to mortality.

Gross (Hospital) Death Rate

In computing hospital death rates, the concept of number of occurrences versus number of times something could have occurred still applies. That is, every patient discharged from the hospital could possibly have died. Of course, this does not happen, but it is still a statistical possibility. Therefore, the formula for calculating the hospital death rate (gross death rate) is the number of patient deaths divided by the number of patient discharges (including deaths), as shown:

$$\frac{\textit{Number of inpatient deaths (including NB) in a period} \times 100}{\textit{Number of discharges (including A\&C and NB deaths) in the same period}}$$

Example: If a hospital had five deaths and 400 discharges for a month, the gross death rate would be:

$$\frac{(5 \times 100)}{400} = 1.25\%$$

This concept can be explored more specifically by means of the formula referred to as the **case fatality rate:**

$$\frac{\textit{Number of people who die of a disease in a specified period} \times 100}{\textit{Number of people who have the disease}}$$

Using the example of patients with influenza, every patient discharged with the diagnosis of influenza has the potential to die. Thus, the formula is:

$$\frac{\textit{Number of patients with influenza who died} \times 100}{\textit{Number of patients discharged with a diagnosis of influenza}}$$

If a hospital had 20 influenza discharges last year and six deaths, the death rate would be:

$$\frac{(6 \times 100)}{20} = 30.00\%$$

If 20 heart transplant patients were discharged and two died, the calculation would be:

$$\frac{(2 \times 100)}{20} = 10.00\%$$

Example: The case fatality rate can be used to examine the death rates by physician. If Dr. Jones discharged 500 patients and 27 died, the formula would be:

$$\frac{(27 \times 100)}{500} = 5.40\%$$

Guidelines for Calculating Death Rates

In calculating death rates, the following guidelines should be considered:

- Death is a type of discharge or **disposition.** Any data representing total discharges include deaths for that period. Thus, deaths are always assumed to be included in the total discharges in the denominator unless otherwise specified.

- If deaths of **newborn** inpatients are included in the numerator, all discharges of newborn inpatients must be included in the denominator. Ordinarily, newborns are included in the gross death rate unless a facility chooses to calculate their death rate separately.

- Patients who are **dead on arrival** (DOA) are not included in the gross death rate because DOAs are not admitted to the hospital.

- Patients who die in the emergency services department are not included in the gross death rate because they were not admitted to the hospital.

- Patients who die in the hospital while outpatients are not included in the gross death rate.

- **Fetal deaths** are not included in the hospital death rate but are calculated separately.

- Because death rates are ordinarily small, the calculation is usually carried out to three decimal places and rounded down to two places.

- It is a good idea to put a zero in front of the decimal (for example, 0.23%) to show the casual observer that the rate is less than 1 percent.

Exercise 6.1

Using the data below, calculate (round to two decimal places) the gross death rate at Community Hospital for May. (Deaths are not included in the discharges.)

Community Hospital
May 20XX Data

Total adult and children live discharges	540
Total adult and children deaths	9
Total newborn live discharges	62
Total newborn deaths	1

Answer:

Exercise 6.2

The table below is a sample report for a hospital showing the discharges and deaths for the last quarter of the year. Notice that this report lists the patient discharges and deaths by physicians on the medical staff. Calculate the death rates for each physician and the total for this quarter (round to two decimal places). Deaths are not included in the discharges.

Community Hospital
October–December 20XX
Discharges and Deaths—Total Hospital Services

Physician Number	No. of Discharges	No. of Deaths	Gross Death Rate
Dr. 097	47	3	
Dr. 123	107	4	
Dr. 256	9	1	
Dr. 372	85	4	
Dr. 431	119	6	
Dr. 537	76	2	
Dr. 638	98	4	
Dr. 725	55	3	
Dr. 800	117	1	
Dr. 901	132	8	
Total			

Handy Tip: You may notice when computing your rates that sometimes your answer may be a whole number, such as 6 percent, or there may be a zero in the hundredths place as in 6.1 percent. When asked to compute to two decimal places, always add the zeros. Your answers would read 6.00 percent and 6.10 percent.

Net Death Rate

Various reporting or accrediting agencies sometimes request the **net death rate,** also referred to as the **institutional death rate.** When calculating the net death rate, newborn deaths are included in the inpatient deaths with the adult/children deaths. Historically, hospital inpatient deaths were classified either as those that occurred less than 48 hours after admission and those deaths that occurred 48 hours or more after admission.

The net death rate came into use because it was felt that healthcare providers should not be held accountable for a death that occurred less than 48 hours after admission because they would not have had enough time to directly affect the patient's condition; only emergency treatment could be provided during this period of time. However, with the technology available today, many authorities believe this concept is no longer valid. Regardless of this consideration, the net death rate excludes deaths under 48 hours and is less than the gross death rate.

The formula for calculating the net death rate is:

$$\frac{\textit{Total number of inpatient deaths (including NB) minus deaths} < 48 \textit{ hours for a given period} \times 100}{\textit{Total number of discharges (including NB deaths) minus deaths} < 48 \textit{ hours from the same period}}$$

Example: Last month, Community Hospital had 155 discharges, including eight deaths. Three of the deaths were patients who were in the hospital less than 48 hours. The net death rate would be calculated as follows:

$$\frac{(8-3)\times100}{(155-3)} = \frac{500}{152} = 3.29\%$$

Exercise 6.3

Using the data in the table below, calculate (round to two decimal places) the net death rate at Community Hospital for October. Discharges do not include deaths.

**Community Hospital
October 20XX Data**

Total adult and children discharges	307
Total adult and children deaths	5
Deaths < 48 hours	1
Deaths ≥ 48 hours	4
Total newborn discharges	62
Total newborn deaths	2
Deaths < 48 hours	1
Deaths ≥ 48 hours	1

Answer:

Exercise 6.4

Using the information in the table below, calculate (round to two decimal places) the net death rate for each service and the total net death rate at Community Hospital for September. In this exercise deaths are included in the discharges.

**Community Hospital
September 20XX Data**

Service	No. of Discharges	Deaths < 48 hours	Deaths ≥ 48 hours	Net Death Rate
Medicine	265	3	7	
Surgery	237	1	2	
Psychiatric	92	1	1	
Rehabilitation	42	1	3	
Total				

Postoperative Death Rate

The **postoperative death rate,** also called the **surgical death rate,** refers to the number of deaths occurring after an operation has been performed. Standard instructions for computing the postoperative death rate involve the ratio of deaths within 10 days after surgery to the total number of patients operated on during that period.

In appendix B of this book, a **surgical operation** is defined as one or more surgical procedures performed at one time for one patient via a common approach or for a common purpose. A **surgical procedure** is any single, separate, systematic process upon or within the body that can be complete in itself; is normally performed by a physician, dentist, or other licensed practitioner; can be performed either with or without instruments; and is performed to restore disunited or deficient parts, remove diseased or injured tissues, extract foreign matter, assist in obstetrical delivery, or aid in diagnosis.

The formula for calculating the postoperative death rate is:

$$\frac{Total \; number \; of \; deaths \; (within \; 10 \; days \; after \; surgery) \times 100}{Total \; number \; of \; patients \; who \; were \; operated \; on \; for \; the \; period}$$

However, some healthcare practitioners question the usefulness of this calculation in evaluating the effectiveness of a hospital's medical care. Thus, rather than compute a total postoperative death rate, some hospitals evaluate the relationship of deaths following specific operations (for example, cholecystectomies or coronary artery bypass grafts).

Handy Tip: The standard formula for a rate applies here as well. All individuals who have surgery have the potential to die. The only difference here is that convention places a time limit of 10 days. After 10 days, concerns other than the surgery may cause the death of a patient. The denominator includes the patients operated on and not the number of operations because one patient may have several operations during a hospital stay.

Exercise 6.5

Using the information in the table below, calculate (round to two decimal places) the postoperative death rate for each surgeon at Community Hospital between January and March.

Community Hospital
January–March 20XX
Number of Surgery Patients and Deaths, by Surgeon

Physician Number	No. of Surgery Patients	No. of Deaths within 10 Days after Surgery	Postoperative Death Rate
Dr. 102	180	4	
Dr. 237	120	2	
Dr. 391	60	1	
Dr. 518	65	1	
Dr. 637	98	5	
Dr. 802	32	3	
Dr. 900	64	1	

Exercise 6.6

Using the information in the table that follows, calculate (round to two decimal places) the postoperative death rate at Community Hospital during April.

Community Hospital
April 20XX Data
Surgery Service

Discharges	376
Deaths	6
Within 10 days after surgery	4
More than 10 days after surgery	2
Number of operations	383
Number of patients operated on	370

Answer:

Exercise 6.7

Using the information in the table below, calculate (round to two decimal places) the postoperative death rate at Community Hospital for each Medicare Severity Diagnosis Related Group (MS-DRG) listed for July through December and the total for this semiannual period.

Community Hospital
July–December 20XX
Selected MS-DRGs—Postoperative Deaths
Number of Surgery Patients and Deaths
Surgery Service

MS-DRG	MS-DRG Title	No. of Surgery Patients	No. of Deaths within 10 Days after Surgery	Postoperative Death Rate
338	Appendectomy w complicated principal diag w MCC	8	1	
327	Stomach, esophageal & duodenal proc w CC	67	2	
005	Liver transplant w MCC or intestinal transplant	17	6	
139	Salivary gland procedures	5	1	
405	Pancreas, liver & shunt procedures w MCC	54	3	
625	Thyroid, parathyroid & thyroglossal procedures w MCC	195	2	
736	Uterine & adnexa proc for ovarian or adnexal malignancy w MCC	132	5	
217	Cardiac valve & oth maj cardiothoracic proc w card cath w CC	201	3	
239	Amputation for circ sys disorders exc upper limb & toe w MCC	8	3	
469	Major joint replacement or reattachment of lower extremity w MCC	132	4	
Total				

Anesthesia Death Rate

The traditional definition of **anesthesia death rate** is the ratio of deaths caused by anesthetic agents during a specified period to the number of anesthetics administered. Because anesthesia deaths occur infrequently, some hospitals might choose, instead, to evaluate the relationship between a death and a specific anesthetic for a special study.

There are three major types of anesthesia: general, regional, and local. General anesthesia puts the entire body to sleep. It is given intravenously or inhaled. Regional anesthesia removes the ability to feel any pain or sensations in a specific region of the body. This generally involves an injection of a local anesthetic agent around major nerves or the spinal cord. Spinal and epidural anesthesia and peripheral nerve blocks are types of regional anesthesia and are used in many operations on specific portions of the body. Local anesthesia numbs a small area of the body. This involves an injection of an anesthetic, in this case, a numbing agent, directly into the area to block pain. During the procedure the patient may also receive medication to help him or her relax.

The formula for calculating the anesthesia death rate is:

$$\frac{Total\ deaths\ caused\ by\ anesthetic\ agents \times 100}{Total\ number\ of\ anesthetics\ administered}$$

Example: If anesthetics were given 3,000 times to surgical patients and one patient death was attributed to anesthesia during the past year, the anesthesia death rate would be computed as follows:

$$\frac{(1 \times 100)}{3,000} = 0.03\%$$

Handy Tip: The fact that anesthesia deaths occur infrequently is reason to always check the placement of the decimal point in calculations of anesthesia death rates.

Exercise 6.8

Using the information in the table below, calculate (round to two decimal places) the anesthesia death rate for University Hospital for July through December.

University Hospital
July–December 20XX
Surgery Service

Discharges	1,326
Deaths:	46
Within 10 days	14
After 10 days	32
Number of operations	1,329
Number of patients operated on	1,320
Number of anesthetics administered	1,326
Number of deaths due to anesthetic agents	4

Answer:

Exercise 6.9

Using the information in the table below, compute individually (round to two decimal places) the number of deaths due to the administration of general, regional, and local anesthesia.

University Hospital
July–December 20XX
Surgery Service

Discharges	1,326
Deaths	46
Within 10 days	14
After 10 days	32
Number of operations	1,329
Number of patients operated on	1,320
Number of anesthetics administered	1,326
General anesthesia	663
Regional anesthesia	530
Local anesthesia	133
Number of deaths due to anesthetic agents	4
General anesthesia	2
Regional anesthesia	1
Local anesthesia	1

Answers:

General anesthesia:

Regional anesthesia:

Local anesthesia:

Maternal Death Rate

A **maternal death** is defined as the death of any woman from any cause related to or aggravated by pregnancy or its management (regardless of duration or site of pregnancy, but not from accidental or incidental causes). An example of an accidental death would be a motor vehicle accident or a fall down a flight of stairs. An example of an incidental death would be a suicide or homicide.

Many healthcare facilities also differentiate between direct obstetric deaths and indirect obstetric deaths. A *direct obstetric death* is a death directly related to the pregnancy, for example, a patient who died after a C-section because of a nick to the uterine artery that resulted in hemorrhage. An *indirect obstetric death* is not directly due to obstetric causes, even though the physiologic effects of the pregnancy are partially responsible for the death. An example of an indirect obstetric death is diabetes. A pregnant woman can have **complications** of the diabetes that are aggravated by the pregnancy, but the cause of death is the diabetes and not the pregnancy.

Computing Maternal Death Rate

When computing the **maternal death rate,** hospitals usually classify only direct obstetric deaths as maternal deaths and include only those deaths that occur during hospitalization. Non-maternal deaths (deaths resulting from accidental or incidental causes not related to pregnancy or its management) are not included. A woman who dies after an abortion is considered a maternal death, as is an obstetric patient who dies in the **prepartum** period (that is, the time period occurring before childbirth—some facilities refer to these as *antepartum* deaths) of a cause due to pregnancy. If the service classification system includes a breakdown of obstetrical discharges into delivered, aborted, not delivered, and **postpartum** (the time after childbirth), all these should be included in the total obstetrical discharges in the denominator of the formula (and in the numerator if the mother dies).

The formula for calculating the maternal death rate is:

$$\frac{\textit{Number of direct maternal deaths for a period} \times 100}{\textit{Number of obstetrical discharges (including deaths) for the period}}$$

Example: At one hospital, a mother died immediately after delivery. The hospital's annual obstetric/gynecology discharges are classified as: delivered, 5,000; aborted, 100; not delivered (prepartum), 200; and postpartum, 20.

Please note in this example that some patients are divided into prepartum (not delivered) and postpartum cases. A patient who comes into the hospital in labor but does not deliver and is discharged home is considered a prepartum patient; a patient who comes into the hospital after delivery with an infection of the C-section incision site is considered a postpartum patient.

The calculation of the hospital maternal mortality rate is:

$$\frac{(1 \times 100)}{(5,000 + 100 + 200 + 20)} = \frac{100}{5,320} = 0.018 = 0.02\%$$

Handy Tip: Just as with other death rates, the maternal death rate calculation is usually carried to three decimal places and then rounded to two places.

Computing Vital Statistics for Maternal Mortality Rate

As previously noted in chapter 1, researchers frequently use vital statistics information for public health and policy studies. Researchers use a number other than 100 in the numerator because they are not interested in determining percentages but, rather, the number of times something occurs in the population. For example, researchers may use 100,000 to determine how often something occurred per 100,000 people, 10,000 to determine how often it occurred per 10,000 people, and so on.

The following vital statistics formula for maternal mortality rate may be used in the United States:

$$\frac{\textit{Number of deaths attributed to maternal conditions during a period} \times 100,000}{\textit{Number of births during the period}}$$

Example: During the year, a community hospital reported 1,205 **hospital live births** and two deaths after abortions. The vital statistics maternal mortality rate would be calculated as follows:

$$\frac{(2 \times 100,000)}{1,205} = \frac{200,000}{1,205} = 165.975 = 166 \text{ per } 100,000 \text{ births}$$

$$\frac{(2 \times 10,000)}{1,205} = \frac{20,000}{1,205} = 16.5975 = 16.6 \text{ per } 10,000 \text{ births}$$

$$\frac{(2 \times 1,000)}{1,205} = \frac{2,000}{1,205} = 1.65 = 1.7 \text{ per } 1,000 \text{ births}$$

Exercise 6.10

Using the information in the table below, calculate (round to two decimal places) Community Hospital's maternal death rate for April. These are all direct maternal deaths.

Community Hospital
April 20XX
Obstetrical Unit

Discharges	
Delivered	220
Aborted	2
Undelivered, prepartum	22
Undelivered, postpartum	15
Deaths	
Delivered	1
Aborted	1
Undelivered, prepartum	1
Undelivered, postpartum	2

Answer:

Exercise 6.11

Last month, The Women's Hospital reported 134 obstetrical discharges and four deaths. (The deaths are included in the discharges.) The causes of the four deaths were:

- Injuries due to abuse by husband
- Heroin overdose
- Hemorrhage after C-section due to severed uterine artery
- Pregnancy-induced hypertension

Calculate the direct maternal death rate (round to two decimal places) for this hospital.

Exercise 6.12

Using the annual statistics in the table below, calculate (round to two decimal places) the maternal death rate and the abortion death rate for University Hospital. These are all direct maternal deaths.

University Hospital
Annual Statistics 20XX
Obstetrical Service

Discharges:

Delivered	903
Aborted	36
Undelivered, prepartum	85
Undelivered, postpartum	76

Deaths:

Delivered	2
Aborted	1
Undelivered, prepartum	1
Undelivered, postpartum	1

Answers:

Maternal death rate:

Abortion death rate:

Another statistic that is used in the description of maternal deaths is one by the **World Health Organization (WHO)**. The WHO describes a maternal death as the death of a woman while pregnant or within 42 days of termination of pregnancy from any cause related to or aggravated by the pregnancy. It includes all pregnancies no matter the length of the pregnancy or the location (uterine or ectopic) of the pregnancy, except those deaths from accidental or incidental causes.

The formula for the WHO maternal mortality rate is as follows:

$$\frac{Number\ of\ maternal\ deaths \times 100,000}{Number\ of\ live\ births}$$

Exercise 6.13

In 2005 there were 4,138,349 live births in the United States. According to the WHO there were 440 documented maternal deaths in the United States. What is the maternal mortality rate per 100,000? Calculate to the nearest whole number.

Newborn Mortality Rate

Statistical tabulations for vital events related to pregnancy and newborns can provide valuable information on reproductive health. They also can provide data on national and international trends.

The following definitions apply to infant deaths:

- **Newborn death** refers to the death of a liveborn infant born in the hospital who later dies during the same admission.

- **Neonatal death** refers to the death of a liveborn infant within the **neonatal period** of 27 days, 23 hours, and 59 minutes from the moment of birth.

- **Postneonatal death** refers to the death of a liveborn infant from 28 days of birth to the end of the first year of life (through 364 days, 23 hours, 59 minutes from the moment of birth).

- **Infant death** refers to the death of a liveborn infant at any time from the moment of birth to the end of the first year of life (through 364 days, 23 hours, 59 minutes from the moment of birth).

- **Perinatal death** is an all-inclusive term referring to both stillborn infants and neonatal deaths.

The formula for calculating the **newborn mortality rate** (also called the **newborn death rate**) is:

$$\frac{Total\ number\ of\ newborn\ deaths\ for\ a\ period \times 100}{Total\ number\ of\ newborn\ discharges\ (including\ deaths)\ for\ the\ period}$$

Handy Tip: When computing newborn mortality rates, the answer should be carried out to at least three decimal places and rounded to two places. This is important because newborn death rates are usually very small. When healthcare facilities report discharges, they typically include deaths in the discharge figures because a death is a type of a discharge.

Example: If University Hospital had 2,000 newborn discharges and one newborn death in one year, its newborn mortality rate would be calculated as:

$$\frac{(1 \times 100)}{2,000} = 0.05\%$$

Computing Vital Statistics for Neonatal and Infant Mortality Rates

Researchers frequently use birth certificate data for public health and policy studies. Similar vital statistics formulas are used in the United States. Following are two examples of vital statistics formulas.

Neonatal mortality rate formula:

$$\frac{Number\ of\ neonatal\ deaths\ during\ a\ period \times 1,000}{Number\ of\ live\ births\ during\ the\ period}$$

Infant mortality rate formula:

$$\frac{Number\ of\ infant\ deaths\ (neonatal\ and\ postneonatal)\ during\ a\ period \times 1,000}{Number\ of\ live\ births\ during\ the\ period}$$

Example: If a hospital had 3,856 births, three newborn deaths, and 3,850 newborn discharges, the vital statistics neonatal mortality rate would be calculated as follows:

$$\frac{(3 \times 1,000)}{3,856} = \frac{3,000}{3,856} = 0.7780 = 0.8\ per\ 1,000$$

Exercise 6.14

1. Using the information in the table below, calculate (round to two decimal places) Community Hospital's annual newborn mortality rate. In this exercise, the deaths are included in the discharges.

Community Hospital
Annual Statistics 20XX
Newborn Service

Births	379
Newborn deaths	1
Newborn discharges	380

Answer:

2. Using the information in the table below, calculate (round to two decimal places) the newborn death rate for February at Community Hospital. In this exercise, the deaths are included in the discharges.

Community Hospital
Newborn Unit
February 20XX

Births	32
Discharges	32
Deaths	1

Answer:

Fetal Death Rate

A hospital fetal death is defined as a death prior to the complete expulsion or extraction from the mother (in a hospital facility) of a product of human conception (fetus and placenta) regardless of the duration of pregnancy. The death is indicated by the fact that after such expulsion or extraction, the fetus does not breathe or show any other evidence of life (for example, beating of the heart, pulsation of the umbilical cord, or definite movement of voluntary muscles). Typically, hospitals are required to report fetal deaths to a state agency. However, the reporting method varies according to individual state laws, statutes, and regulations.

Because fetal deaths are not considered patient deaths, they are not included in any other calculation of deaths but, instead, are calculated separately. Determination of whether to include fetal death data in a specific hospital's statistics requires an investigation of the facility's needs by hospital administration, medical staff, and reporting agencies. Fetal deaths are classified as:

- **Early fetal death:** Fewer than 20 weeks of gestation and a weight of 500 grams or less

- **Intermediate fetal death:** Twenty completed weeks of gestation (but less than 28 weeks) and a weight of 501 to 1,000 grams

- **Late fetal death:** Twenty-eight completed weeks of gestation and a weight of 1,001 grams or more

Both intermediate and late fetal deaths constitute what is commonly termed a **stillbirth.** The formula for calculating the **fetal death rate** is:

$$\frac{Total\ number\ of\ intermediate\ and/or\ late\ fetal\ deaths\ for\ a\ period \times 100}{Total\ number\ of\ live\ births\ +\ Intermediate\ and\ late\ fetal\ deaths\ for\ the\ period}$$

Example: During June, a hospital had 100 live births, one intermediate fetal death, and three late fetal deaths. To determine the fetal death rate for the hospital, the total number of intermediate and late fetal deaths (4) is multiplied by 100 and divided by the total number of live births and the intermediate and late fetal deaths (100 + 4). The calculation is as follows:

$$\frac{(4 \times 100)}{(100 + 4)} = \frac{400}{104} = 3.846\% = 3.85\%$$

Handy Tip: Keep in mind that the denominator in the fetal death rate formula does not include discharges. If you remember the formula for rates discussed in chapter 2, that is, the number of times something actually happened in relation to the number of times it could have happened, it becomes clear that every birth could be a fetal death. And, be sure to include the intermediate and late fetal deaths in the denominator.

Handy Tip: Also remember that newborn births are the same as newborn admissions.

Exercise 6.15

Community Hospital reported the following statistics for the month of July. Calculate (round to two decimal places) the fetal death rate.

**Community Hospital
July 20XX
Newborn Service**

Live births	29
Newborn discharges	32
Fetal deaths:	
Early	1
Intermediate	2
Late	4

Answer:

Exercise 6.16

Using the information in the table below, calculate (round to two decimal places) the newborn mortality rate and fetal death rate at Community Hospital for the year. In this exercise, deaths are included in the discharges.

**Community Hospital
January–December 20XX
Newborn Service**

Live births	245
Newborn discharges	248
Newborn deaths	3
Fetal deaths:	
Early	5
Intermediate	3
Late	1

Answers:
Newborn death rate:

Fetal death rate:

Cancer Mortality Rate

A **mortality rate** measures the risk of death for the cause under study in a defined population during a given time period. The National Center for Health Statistics collects data on all cancer deaths occurring in the United States and classifies them by sex, age, race, and cancer site so that mortality for a given time period can be determined for the entire country or selected areas.

The formula for calculating the **cancer mortality rate** for a population is:

$$\frac{Number\ of\ cancer\ deaths\ during\ a\ period \times 100,000}{Total\ number\ in\ population\ at\ risk}$$

Example: In 2007, 562,875 people died from cancer in the United States. The estimated 2007 census for the US population was 301,621,157. The formula for calculating the cancer mortality rate per 100,000 people in 2007 would be:

$$\frac{Number\ of\ cancer\ deaths\ in\ 2007}{Population\ at\ risk}$$

Using the statistics provided here, the calculation would be as follows:

$$\frac{(562,875 \times 100,000)}{301,621,157} = 186.6\ deaths\ per\ 100,000\ population$$

This is a **crude death rate** because it encompasses deaths from all forms of cancer for persons of all ages and races and of both sexes. In other words, it is based on the entire US population. Specific rates can be calculated to describe risks for specific cancers in entire populations or specific subgroups of a population, such as age-specific rates or sex-specific rates.

Knowledge of healthcare statistics is an essential tool for cancer registrars. A cancer registrar is an individual who is responsible for maintaining records and reporting information about cancer patients. Hospital cancer registries were developed as organized programs in hospitals to collect information about cancer patients. Their primary goal is to help improve treatment of cancer. The information collected can be used to compare different types of therapies used to treat cancer. Hospital and other cancer registry data are reported to population-based (central or regional) registries.

When you are calculating the cancer death rate in your own facility, use the formula for a rate—that is the number of deaths from a specific diagnosis of cancer divided by the number of discharges of that same diagnosis of cancer.

Exercise 6.17

Using the information given in the table below from Community Hospital's Cancer Registry, calculate (round to two decimal places) the death rates for each type of cancer and the total for this annual period. Deaths are included in the discharges.

Community Hospital
Cancer Registry Annual Report
Selected Cancers Reported
20XX

Type of Cancer	No. of Discharges	No. of Deaths	Death Rate
Prostate	23	6	
Breast	56	4	
Lung and bronchus	28	9	
Colon/Rectum	39	2	
Uterus	36	5	
Urinary bladder	15	2	
Non-Hodgkin's lymphoma	21	6	
Melanoma of the skin	23	5	
Kidney and renal pelvis	15	3	
Ovary	12	5	
Total			

Exercise 6.18

Using the statistics in the table below from a multihospital system, calculate (round to two decimal places) the gross death rate for each hospital listed and for the entire healthcare system. In this exercise, the deaths are included in the discharges.

Community Healthcare System
Annual Statistics 20XX

Hospital	Discharges	Deaths	Death Rate
Urban Hospital	14,962	172	
Rural Hospital	5,403	107	
Psychiatric Hospital	1,243	6	
Rehabilitation Hospital	1,159	24	
Total			

Chapter 6 Test

Using the data reported below for the past year, perform the calculations requested below. (Round these to two decimal places.)

Discharges (includes deaths)

Total adults and children	12,954
Total newborns	1,865

The following are included in the discharges:

OB delivered	1,871
OB aborted	125
OB undelivered, prepartum	20
OB undelivered, postpartum	32

Deaths

Total adults and children	47
Total newborns	2

The following are included in the deaths:

Within 10 days postop	2
< 48 hours after admission	12
≥ 48 hours after admission	35
Anesthetic death	1

Obstetric deaths:

Undelivered, prepartum	1
Aborted	1

Fetal deaths:

Early	7
Intermediate	5
Late	2

Admissions

Total adults and children	13,023
Total live births	1,864

Total patients operated on	4,533
Total anesthetics administered	4,533

1. The gross death rate is:
   a. 0.033%
   b. 0.33%
   c. 3.31%
   d. 33.10

2. The net death rate is:
   a. 0.25%
   b. 2.51%
   c. 0.025%
   d. 25.10%

3. The postoperative death rate is 0.05 percent. True or false?

4. What is the anesthesia death rate?

5. What is the maternal death rate?

6. What is the newborn mortality rate?

Chapter 6 Test (continued)

7. What is the fetal death rate?

8. The gross death rate excludes deaths that occur within 48 hours of admission. True or false?

9. According to standard instructions, deaths within 15 days after surgery are used to compute the postoperative death rate. True or false?

10. Anesthesia deaths occur frequently. True or false?

11. Which of the following deaths is also called the institutional death rate?
    a. Gross death rate
    b. Net death rate
    c. Postoperative death rate

12. Define the gestational age and gram weight for early fetal death, intermediate fetal death, and late fetal death.

Use the information in the table below to answer questions 13 through 19. In these exercises, the deaths are included in the discharges; this includes deaths occurring in less than 48 hours and postoperative deaths.

Community Hospital
Annual Statistics 20XX

Service	Discharges	Deaths	< 48 hours	Postop
Medicine	1,375	84	13	0
Surgery	1,098	22	9	3
Obstetrics	632	1	0	0
Newborn	633	1	1	0
Psychiatric	321	1	0	0
Rehabilitation	291	16	0	0
Total				

Additional Information

Anesthetics administered	1,094
Anesthetic deaths	1
Patients operated on	1,094
Total livebirths	633
Fetal deaths:	
Early	7
Intermediate	4
Late	1

(continued on next page)

Chapter 6 Test (continued)

13. What is the gross death rate?

14. What is the net death rate?

15. What is the postoperative death rate?

16. What is the anesthesia death rate?

17. What is the maternal death rate?

18. What is the newborn mortality rate?

19. What is the fetal death rate?

Using the information in the table below, calculate the death rates for University Hospital's Cancer Registry for each of the cancers reported and the total for this annual period. In this exercise, the deaths are included in the discharges.

**University Hospital
Cancer Registry Annual Report
Selected Cancers Reported
20XX**

Type of Cancer	No. of Discharges	No. of Deaths	Death Rate
Prostate	236	16	
Breast	368	24	
Lung and bronchus	281	29	
Colon/Rectum	397	12	
Uterus	130	5	
Urinary bladder	101	2	
Non-Hodgkin's lymphoma	203	16	
Melanoma of the skin	239	5	
Kidney and renal pelvis	105	13	
Ovary	98	15	
Total			

Chapter 7
Hospital Autopsies and Autopsy Rates

Key Terms

Adjusted hospital autopsy rate

Autopsy

Autopsy rate

Available for hospital autopsy

Coroner

Coroner's case

Fetal autopsy rate

Gross autopsy rate

Hospital autopsy

Hospital autopsy rate

Hospital inpatient autopsy

Medical examiner

Morgue

Necropsy

Net autopsy rate

Newborn autopsy rate

Postmortem examination

Objectives

At the conclusion of this chapter, you should be able to:

- Define the terms autopsy, hospital inpatient autopsy, hospital autopsy, and autopsy rate

- Define and differentiate between a coroner and medical examiner

- Define a coroner's case and determine when it would be included in a hospital's autopsy rate

- Compute the following autopsy rates: gross, net, adjusted hospital, newborn, and fetal

Autopsy

An **autopsy** is the examination of a dead body to determine the cause of death. Autopsies are performed in order to educate physicians and allied health professionals. An autopsy can be performed on the entire body or a particular body organ. Another name for autopsy is **necropsy** or **postmortem** (after death) **examination.** Autopsies are generally performed by either a hospital pathologist or a physician on the medical staff who has been delegated this responsibility. They are usually performed in the hospital **morgue,** but in the case of small hospitals that do not have a morgue, the body may be removed to an off-site lab or a funeral home for the autopsy.

Gross Autopsy Rate

The **autopsy rate** is the proportion of deaths that are followed by the performance of an autopsy. A **gross autopsy rate** is the ratio during any given period of time of all inpatient autopsies to all inpatient deaths. The rate is customarily reported as a percentage. Again, the concept of a rate applies here: the number of times something actually happened compared to the number of times it could have happened. Statistically speaking, every patient who died could be autopsied. Typically, newborn autopsies are included in the gross autopsy rate but may be calculated separately as determined by the hospital's administration or medical staff committee.

The formula for calculating the gross autopsy rate is:

$$\frac{Total\ autopsies\ on\ inpatient\ deaths\ for\ a\ period \times 100}{Total\ inpatient\ deaths\ for\ the\ period}$$

Example: During July, University Hospital discharged 819 patients. The hospital had 24 deaths (including newborns) and performed 9 autopsies. Using the formula given above, the gross autopsy rate is determined to be 37.50 percent, as follows:

$$\frac{(9 \times 100)}{24} = \frac{900}{24} = 37.50\%$$

Handy Tip: Although death rates are usually small, autopsy rates can be fairly large.

Exercise 7.1

In a one-month period, a 360-bed hospital with 20 bassinets reported 24 inpatient deaths. The medical staff performed 6 autopsies. The gross autopsy rate is 32.50 percent. True or false?

Exercise 7.2

Using the information in the table below, calculate (round to two decimal places) the gross death rate, the net death rate, and the gross autopsy rate for Community Hospital for the time period.

Community Hospital
Hospital Statistics
January–June 20XX

Total inpatient discharges (including deaths)	378
Total inpatient deaths	18
(< 48 hours—included in total inpatient deaths)	(3)
Total autopsies	5

Answers:

Gross death rate:

Net death rate:

Gross autopsy rate:

Net Autopsy Rate

The **net autopsy rate** is the ratio during any given period of time of all inpatient autopsies to all inpatient deaths, minus any unautopsied coroners' or medical examiners' cases. The formula for net autopsy rate differs slightly from the formula for gross autopsy rate in that it excludes bodies that have been removed by the coroner or medical examiner.

Certain types of deaths are reportable to the coroner of a particular jurisdiction. A **coroner** is the official (elected or appointed, physician or nonphysician) who is responsible for determining the cause, time, and manner of death in unattended, violent, or unexplained deaths. Coroners may also have other duties depending on their state. The word comes from the Old English word *corono,* which means "crown." The English crown originally appointed coroners.

In some areas of the country, the coroner has been replaced with a **medical examiner** (ME). The medical examiner is usually an appointed official who is a physician, commonly holding a specialty in pathology or forensic medicine. A body released to a coroner or medical examiner is not available for autopsy by the hospital pathologist.

The formula for calculating the net autopsy rate is:

$$\frac{Total\ autopsies\ on\ inpatient\ deaths\ for\ a\ period \times 100}{Total\ inpatient\ deaths - Unautopsied\ coroners'\ or\ medical\ examiners'\ cases}$$

Example: During January, Community Hospital had 12 patient deaths and performed 5 autopsies. Two bodies were released to the county coroner for autopsy. Therefore, two cases are subtracted from the denominator because they were not autopsied by the hospital. Dividing the number of inpatient autopsies performed (5) by the total number of bodies available for autopsy (12 – 2 = 10) produces a net autopsy rate of 50 percent, as shown in the equation below.

$$\frac{(5 \times 100)}{(12-2)} = \frac{500}{10} = 50.0\%$$

Handy Tip: If the coroner or medical examiner requests the hospital pathologist perform the autopsy, it is included in the rate and not subtracted out because the case would not be unavailable for autopsy.

Exercise 7.3

Over the past year, University Hospital had 16,523 discharges, 288 inpatient deaths, and 185 autopsies. The bodies of 20 patients were released to the medical examiner for autopsy. Calculate (round to two decimal places) the gross death, gross autopsy, and net autopsy rates for University Hospital.

Answers:

Gross death rate:

Gross autopsy rate:

Net autopsy rate:

Handy Tip: The net autopsy rate will be higher than the gross autopsy rate because the denominator includes unautopsied coroners' or medical examiners' cases. Because there is a lower number of autopsies in the denominator, the rate will be higher.

Exercise 7.4

Using the information in the table below, calculate (round to two decimal places) the gross death, gross autopsy, and net autopsy rates for University Hospital. In this exercise, the deaths are included in the discharges.

University Hospital
Quarterly Statistics
October–December 20XX

Discharges:	
Adults and children	3,304
Newborn	826
Deaths:	
Adults and children	70
Newborn	2
Inpatient autopsies	46
Coroner's cases (unavailable for autopsy)	5

Answers:

Gross death rate:

Gross autopsy rate:

Net autopsy rate:

Hospital Autopsies

A **hospital inpatient autopsy** is the postmortem examination that is ordinarily performed in a hospital facility on the body of an inpatient who died during hospitalization. In contrast, a **hospital autopsy** is the postmortem examination of the body of a person who has *at some time* been a hospital patient. Former inpatients may include emergency patients, outpatients, and home care patients.

When determining what autopsies to include in the **hospital autopsy rate,** the following guidelines apply:

- Hospital autopsies are usually performed by the facility pathologist. However, small hospitals do not always have a pathologist on staff, so responsibility for performing autopsies may be delegated to another physician.

- Normally, hospital autopsies are performed in hospitals. However, a small hospital or a specialized hospital (for example, obstetrical or psychiatric) may not have many deaths and thus may not be equipped with the necessary facilities to perform autopsies. In such cases, the autopsies are performed in another designated place.

- As a general rule, hospital autopsies are performed on inpatients who have died. However, because of the educational value of autopsies, former inpatients who were not in the hospital at the time of death may be considered for hospital autopsies. These individuals may include Emergency Services Department (ESD) patients, outpatients, and home care or hospice deaths. This is the only case where outpatients are included with inpatient statistics.

- Fetal autopsies are not included in the hospital autopsy rate because a fetus is not considered a patient.

- The essential components for a hospital autopsy are the following:

  — The autopsy must be performed by a staff pathologist or a delegated physician.

  — There must be a consent from the patient's next of kin or legal representative to perform an autopsy, which is filed in the medical record. The consent may be for a full body autopsy or a partial autopsy.

  — The autopsy report must be filed in the patient's health record.

  — The tissue specimens must be filed in the hospital laboratory along with the autopsy report.

Examples of hospital autopsy cases include:

- A patient dies in the hospital and is autopsied by the hospital's pathologist in the local morgue.

- A patient dies in the hospital, and one of the hospital's physicians is delegated to perform the autopsy in the absence of the staff pathologist.

- A former patient is pronounced dead on arrival (DOA) in the hospital's ESD, and the staff pathologist performs the autopsy.

Adjusted Hospital Autopsy Rate

The **adjusted hospital autopsy rate** is the proportion of hospital autopsies performed following the deaths of patients whose bodies are available for autopsy. Although many hospitals calculate the net autopsy rate for various surveys and external reports, the adjusted hospital autopsy rate is a more accurate indication of the hospital's resources for physician education because it includes all autopsies.

The formula for calculating the adjusted hospital autopsy rate is:

$$\frac{\textit{Total hospital autopsies} \times 100}{\textit{Total number of deaths of hospital patients whose bodies are available for autopsy}}$$

Patients whose bodies are **available for hospital autopsy** include:

- Inpatients (unless the bodies are removed from the hospital by legal authorities such as the coroner or medical examiner). However, if the hospital pathologist or delegated physician performs an autopsy while acting as an agent of the coroner or medical examiner, the autopsy is included in the numerator and the death in the denominator of the adjusted hospital autopsy rate formula.

- Other patients, including hospital home care patients, outpatients, and previous hospital patients who have died elsewhere and whose bodies have been made available for the performance of hospital autopsies.

Example: Community Hospital had 255 discharges in July, eight of which were deaths. The hospital pathologist performed three of the autopsies. During this period, two home care patients died and were brought to the hospital for autopsy. To determine the adjusted hospital autopsy rate, add all the hospital autopsies performed to determine the numerator (3 inpatients + 2 home care patients). The denominator contains all the inpatients and home care patients who died in July (8 + 2).

$$\frac{(3+2) \times 100}{(8+2)} = 50.0\%$$

Handy Tip: In the previous formulas, outpatients, ESD patients, and home care patients were not included with the inpatients. When calculating the adjusted hospital autopsy rate, the outpatients, ESD patients, and home care patients would be included if their bodies were autopsied by the hospital pathologist.

Exercise 7.5

Community General Hospital had 27 inpatient deaths, 11 of which were autopsied. Two of the 27 deaths were coroner's cases, but one was autopsied by the hospital pathologist. In addition, the following bodies were brought to the hospital for autopsy: three former patients who died in the ER, two former inpatients who died in a skilled nursing facility, one former inpatient who died at home, and one patient who died during a round of outpatient chemotherapy. What is the adjusted hospital autopsy rate? Round to two decimal places.

Exercise 7.6

Using the data in the table below, calculate (round to two decimal places) the gross death, gross autopsy, net autopsy, and adjusted hospital autopsy rates for University Hospital. In this exercise, the deaths are included in the discharges.

University Hospital
Annual Statistics
20XX

Discharges:	
Adults and children	12,924
Newborn	4,332
Deaths:	
Adults and children	345
Newborn	3
Deaths in the ESD and OPD*	15
Autopsies:	
Inpatient	159
ESD/OPD	14
Coroner's cases (unavailable for autopsy)	6

Answers:

Gross death rate:

Gross autopsy rate:

Net autopsy rate:

Adjusted hospital autopsy rate:

---

*ESD = Emergency Services Department; OPD = Outpatient Department

Exercise 7.7

Using the information in the table below, calculate (round to two decimal places) the adjusted hospital autopsy rate.

Community Hospital
July Statistics

Inpatient deaths	8
ESD deaths	3
Home health death	1
Inpatient autopsies	2
ESD autopsy	1
Home health autopsy	1
Coroner's case (unavailable for autopsy)	1

Answer:

Adjusted hospital autopsy rate:

Exercise 7.8

In January, University Hospital had 23 inpatient deaths, eight of which were autopsied. Of the 23 deaths, two were coroner's cases—one of which was autopsied by the hospital pathologist (included in the eight autopsies) and one removed to be autopsied by the coroner. In addition, the following cases were brought to the hospital to be autopsied: a former inpatient who died in a skilled nursing facility a month after discharge from the hospital, a child known to have congenital heart disease who died in the ESD, one patient who died in the outpatient department while he was getting lab work performed, and a former inpatient who died at home while under the hospital's home care department. Calculate (round to two decimal places) the adjusted hospital autopsy rate for University Hospital for this month.

Newborn Autopsy Rate

The **newborn autopsy rate** is the proportion of hospital autopsies performed following the deaths of newborns.

The formula for calculating the newborn autopsy rate is:

$$\frac{Newborn\ autopsies\ for\ a\ period \times 100}{Total\ newborn\ deaths\ for\ the\ period}$$

Example: Community Hospital had 27 births during the month of September. One newborn died shortly after birth and was autopsied. Applying the formula above, the correct newborn autopsy rate is 100 percent.

$$\frac{(1 \times 100)}{1} = 100.0\%$$

Exercise 7.9

Using the information in the table below, calculate (round to two decimal places) the newborn death rate and the newborn autopsy rate for University Hospital. In this exercise, the deaths are included in the discharges.

University Hospital
Newborn Statistics

Births	402
Discharges	398
Deaths	3
Autopsies	2

Answers:

Newborn death rate:

Newborn autopsy rate:

Exercise 7.10

In September 20XX, the newborn unit at Community Hospital reported four stillbirths and two newborn deaths. An autopsy was performed on one of the newborns and two stillbirths. Calculate (round to two decimal places) the newborn autopsy rate for September.

Answer:

Newborn autopsy rate:

Exercise 7.11

University Hospital reported the following quarterly statistics for January–March 20XX: 483 newborn discharges, four newborn deaths, three stillbirths. There were two newborn autopsies. One newborn was born in a taxi on the way to the hospital, was admitted, and later died. It was autopsied. One newborn was born at home and brought to the hospital and admitted. It also died and was autopsied. Calculate (round to two decimal places) University Hospital's newborn death rate and newborn autopsy rate. In this exercise, the deaths are included in the discharges.

Answers:

Newborn death rate:

Newborn autopsy rate:

Handy Tip: Remember that a newborn is an inpatient who was born in a hospital at the beginning of the current inpatient hospitalizations. A newborn born outside the hospital and then admitted is considered a pediatric admission.

Fetal Autopsy Rate

The **fetal autopsy rate** is the proportion of hospital autopsies performed following the deaths of intermediate and late fetal deaths.

The formula for the fetal autopsy rate is:

$$\frac{Autopsies\ performed\ on\ intermediate\ and\ late\ fetal\ deaths\ for\ a\ period \times 100}{Total\ intermediate\ and\ late\ fetal\ deaths\ for\ the\ same\ period}$$

Example: A hospital newborn service reported 12 fetal deaths last quarter: six early, four intermediate, and two late. Of these, the two late fetal deaths and one intermediate fetal death were autopsied. Applying the formula above, the fetal autopsy rate for this hospital is 50.00 percent.

$$\frac{[(2\ late\ fetal\ death\ autopsies + 1\ intermediate\ fetal\ death\ autopsy) \times 100]}{(4 + 2)} = 50.00\%$$

Exercise 7.12

Using the information in the table below, calculate (round to two decimal places) the newborn death, fetal death, newborn autopsy, and fetal autopsy rates for the Newborn Service at University Hospital. In this exercise, the newborn deaths are included in the newborn discharges.

University Hospital
Newborn Service Statistics
January–June 20XX

Births	622
Discharges	620
Newborn deaths	3
Newborn autopsies	1
Fetal deaths:	
Early	6
Intermediate	4
Late	2
Fetal death autopsies:	
Early	1
Intermediate	1
Late	1

Answers:

Newborn death rate:

Fetal death rate:

Newborn autopsy rate:

Fetal autopsy rate:

Exercise 7.13

Community Healthcare System reported the statistics in the table below for its four facilities during its past semiannual period. Calculate (round to two decimal places) the newborn death, fetal death, newborn autopsy, and fetal autopsy rates for each facility and for the system as a whole. In this exercise, the deaths are included in the discharges.

**Community Healthcare System
Newborn Statistics
July–December 20XX**

	Urban Hospital	Suburban Hospital	Rural Hospital	Specialty Hospital
Live births	240	235	165	198
Newborn discharges	239	230	162	195
Newborn deaths	2	1	2	16
Fetal deaths:				
Early	5	2	1	7
Intermediate	3	3	1	6
Late	2	1	1	5
Autopsies:				
Newborn	1	0	1	6
Fetal (late and intermediate)	2	1	2	7

Answers:

Urban Hospital
Newborn death rate:

Fetal death rate:

Newborn autopsy rate:

Fetal autopsy rate:

(continued on next page)

Exercise 7.13 (continued)

Suburban Hospital
Newborn death rate:

Fetal death rate:

Newborn autopsy rate:

Fetal autopsy rate:

Rural Hospital
Newborn death rate:

Fetal death rate:

Newborn autopsy rate:

Fetal autopsy rate:

Specialty Hospital
Newborn death rate:

Fetal death rate:

Newborn autopsy rate:

Fetal autopsy rate:

Exercise 7.13 (continued)

System as a Whole
Newborn death rate:

Fetal death rate:

Newborn autopsy rate:

Fetal autopsy rate:

Chapter 7 Test

(Calculate all rates to two decimal places.)

Community Hospital reported the statistics in the table below. Using these data, calculate the rates requested and select the correct calculation for each.

**Community Hospital
Annual Statistics 20XX**

Inpatient discharges:	
Adults and children	7,356
Newborn	730
Inpatient deaths (included in discharges):	
Adults and children	60
Newborn	2
Fetal deaths:	
Early	6
Intermediate	3
Late	2
Inpatient autopsies:	
Adults and children	12
Newborn	2
Coroner's cases:	
Unavailable for autopsy	3
Autopsy by hospital pathologist (included in inpatient autopsies)	1
Fetal death autopsies:	
Intermediate and late	3
Former hospital patient brought in for autopsy	1

(continued on next page)

Chapter 7 Test (continued)

1. Gross autopsy rate

   a. 22.00%
   b. 22.58%
   c. 0.22%
   d. 2.25%

2. Net autopsy rate

   a. 23.73%
   b. 22.58%
   c. 2.37%
   d. 0.23%

3. Adjusted hospital autopsy rate

   a. 23.73%
   b. 23.81%
   c. 25.00%
   d. 0.23%

4. What is the newborn autopsy rate?

5. What is the fetal autopsy rate?

Using the data reported by University Hospital for June 20XX in the table below, calculate the rates (round to two decimal places).

**University Hospital
June 20XX
Statistics**

Discharges:	
Total adults and children	1,166
Newborn	132
Total live births	135
Deaths (included in discharges):	
Adults and children	198
Newborn	5
Autopsies:	
Adults and children	20
Newborn	4
Hospital autopsied outpatients	7
Coroner's cases (unavailable for autopsy)	3
Fetal deaths:	
Early	2
Intermediate	3
Late	2
Fetal death autopsies:	
Intermediate and late	3

Chapter 7 Test (continued)

6. Gross death rate

7. Gross autopsy rate

8. Net autopsy rate

9. Adjusted hospital autopsy rate

10. Newborn autopsy rate

11. Fetal death rate

12. Fetal autopsy rate

13. Using the data in the table below, calculate the gross death, gross autopsy, and net autopsy rates for each month and the year for University Hospital.

University Hospital
Annual Statistics
20XX

Month	Discharges	Inpatient Deaths	Autopsies	Coroner's Cases	Gross Death Rate	Gross Autopsy Rate	Net Autopsy Rate
January	601	5	1	1			
February	585	5	1	2			
March	620	8	6	1			
April	660	2	1	0			
May	621	6	2	1			
June	612	6	3	2			
July	592	9	5	3			
August	589	3	2	0			
September	587	5	2	1			
October	601	6	3	1			
November	611	3	1	0			
December	585	2	1	1			
Total							

(continued on next page)

Chapter 7 Test (continued)

14. Which of the following represents a hospital autopsy? List as many letters as apply.

   a. A former inpatient died at home a month after discharge from the hospital, and his body was brought to the hospital for autopsy.
   b. The coroner authorized the hospital pathologist to perform an autopsy on a patient who died in the ESD after a car accident.
   c. A patient who had been receiving radiation therapy on an outpatient basis at the hospital died at home; her body was brought to the hospital for autopsy.
   d. A victim of gunshot wounds who died in the ESD was autopsied by the medical examiner.
   e. A cardiac patient died in the ESD, and the hospital pathologist performed the autopsy.
   f. The hospital pathologist designated a physician to cover for her while she was away. The physician performed an autopsy on a deceased hospital inpatient.
   g. A late fetal death (stillbirth) was autopsied by the hospital pathologist.

15. What is the principal difference between net autopsy rate and adjusted hospital autopsy rate?

   a. Fetal deaths are not counted in hospital autopsy rates.
   b. Hospital autopsy rates include only those deaths where the bodies are available for autopsy.
   c. The net autopsy rate considers only inpatient deaths.
   d. Legal cases sometimes are excluded from deaths when computing net autopsy rate.

16. The hospital pathologist or some other designated physician is generally the individual allowed to perform autopsies. True or false?

17. In which of the following rates are outpatients who were autopsied counted in an autopsy rate?

   a. Gross autopsy rate
   b. Net autopsy rate
   c. Adjusted hospital autopsy rate
   d. Newborn autopsy rate

18. Why are fetal deaths never counted in any autopsy rate except the fetal autopsy rate?

Chapter 7 Test (continued)

Indicate whether the statements below are true or false. If an answer is false, explain why.

19. To be considered a hospital autopsy, an autopsy must be performed by the staff pathologist or a physician delegated the responsibility.

20. A hospital autopsy must be performed in the hospital.

21. Hospital autopsies are performed only on inpatients.

22. Autopsies on fetuses are included in hospital autopsies.

23. The essentials of a hospital autopsy are that it be performed by the hospital pathologist or a physician delegated the responsibility, there is a consent from the patient's next of kin or legal representative, that an autopsy report be filed in the patient's health record, and that tissue specimens and the autopsy report be filed in the hospital laboratory.

24. The net autopsy rate includes both inpatients and out-of-hospital patients.

25. A deceased hospital inpatient whose body is released to legal authorities for autopsy is not included in the computation of the net autopsy rate.

Chapter 8
Morbidity and Other Miscellaneous Rates

Key Terms

Cesarean-section rate

Chronic

Clean surgical case

Complication

Concomitant

Consultation

Consultation rate

Delivery

Iatrogenic

Infection rate

Morbidity

Nosocomial infection

Nosocomial infection rate

Postoperative infection rate

Objectives

At the conclusion of this chapter, you should be able to:

- Define nosocomial infection

- Discuss and calculate infection rate

- Define and calculate the postoperative infection rate

- Distinguish between a surgical procedure and a surgical operation

- Define complication and calculate complication rate

- When provided with appropriate data, compute the following rates: C-section, consultation, and other rates

Infection Rate

The term **morbidity** means the state of being diseased or the number of sick persons or cases of disease in relation to a specific population. Morbidity may be infectious or have other causes. For example, the presence of **concomitant** (taking place at the same time), **chronic** (of long duration) conditions may constitute comorbidity. Moreover, morbidity may be preexisting (occurring prior to admission to the hospital) or **iatrogenic** (occurring because of the patient's treatment).

Preventing morbidity due to infection is an important quality management function. Frequently, the healthcare facility establishes a committee whose primary function is to evaluate infections and determine their causes so that recurrence can be avoided. Typically called the Infection Prevention Committee, it is composed of representatives from medical staff, nursing, pharmacy, risk management, and health information management. Charged with the duty of infection prevention, committee members establish procedures for the management and reporting of infections. Effective management of infections acquired in the hospital (**nosocomial infections**) sometimes requires finding cases beyond the infections listed by physicians in the medical record. The HIM practitioner can help identify such cases in the course of performing qualitative analysis and coding.

In 1970, the Centers for Disease Control and Prevention (CDC) developed the National Nosocomial Infections Surveillance (NNIS) System to monitor the incidence of nosocomial infections. These may also be referred to as healthcare-associated infections (HAIs). This is a voluntary reporting system and is the only national system for tracking nosocomial infections (CDC 2005). In 2008, the CDC's Division of Healthcare Quality Promotion developed the National Healthcare Safety Network (NHSN) which includes the previous work of the NNIS. "The NHSN is a secure, internet-based surveillance system that integrates former CDC surveillance systems, including the National Nosocomial Infections Surveillance System (NNIS), National Surveillance System for Healthcare Workers (NaSH), and the Dialysis Surveillance Network (DSN). NHSN enables healthcare facilities to collect and use data about healthcare-associated infections, adherence to clinical practices known to prevent healthcare-associated infections, the incidence or prevalence of multidrug-resistant organisms within their organizations, trends and coverage of healthcare personnel safety and vaccination, and adverse events related to the transfusion of blood and blood products." (CDC, 2010)

As defined in chapter 2, the term *rate* refers to the number of times something happened compared to the number of times it could have happened (Rate = Part/Base or R = P/B). Each healthcare facility's medical staff must determine the criteria for inclusion of a patient in both the numerator (infection) and denominator (patients at risk of infection).

Most healthcare facilities differentiate between nosocomial infections and exacerbation and recurrence of previous infections. For example, if an obstetrical patient develops a urinary tract infection, a physician must determine whether it was hospital-acquired or due to a recurrence of a previous urinary tract infection. Most Infection Prevention Departments are more interested in determining whether nosocomial infections are attributable to specific patient care units (PCUs), specific operations, patients with specified diseases, the organized medical staff units, or individual physicians or hospital employees.

The **nosocomial infection rate** is the number of hospital-acquired infections in the hospital for a given time period divided by the total number of inpatient discharges (including deaths) for the same time period.

The formula for calculating the nosocomial infection rate is:

$$\frac{Total\ number\ of\ nosocomial\ infections\ for\ a\ period \times 100}{Total\ number\ of\ discharges,\ including\ deaths,\ for\ the\ same\ period}$$

Example: In January, Community Hospital had 350 discharges and deaths. Thirteen of these patients had hospital-acquired infections. The nosocomial infection rate is 3.7%.

$$\frac{(13 \times 100)}{350} = 3.7\%$$

Infection rates may be calculated separately for specific infections such as surgical wound infections, puerperal infections (infections that occur immediately after childbirth), and infections of the respiratory tract, urinary tract, bloodstream, and so on.

The formula for calculating the infection rate is:

$$\frac{Total\ number\ of\ infections \times 100}{Total\ number\ of\ discharges\ (including\ deaths)\ for\ the\ period}$$

Example: In July, Community Hospital had 150 discharges, eight of whom developed a urinary tract infection while in the hospital. The infection rate is calculated by placing the number of infections (8) × 100 in the numerator and dividing by the 150 (discharges) in the denominator.

$$\frac{(8 \times 100)}{150} = 5.33\%$$

Exercise 8.1

Based on the information in the table below, calculate (round to two decimal places) the rates requested for Community Hospital. In this exercise, deaths are included in the discharges.

**Community Hospital
Annual Statistics
20XX**

Discharges:	
Adults and children	1,784
Newborn	123
Deaths:	
Adults and children	12
Newborn	1
Nosocomial infections:	
Adults and children	13
Newborn	3

Answers:

Nosocomial infection rate for adults and children:

Nosocomial infection rate for newborns:

Total nosocomial infection rate for the hospital:

Gross death rate for this annual period:

Exercise 8.2

Based on the information given in the table below, calculate (round to two decimal places) the rates requested. In this exercise, the deaths are included in the discharges.

University Hospital
Semiannual Statistics
January–June 20XX

Service	No. of Discharges	No. of Deaths	No. of Nosocomial Infections
Medicine	2,333	212	28
Surgery	2,532	102	32
Obstetrics	623	2	3
Psychiatry	452	1	3
Rehabilitation	987	14	19
Pediatrics	832	1	2
Newborn	625	0	2
Total			

Answers:

Gross death rate for each service:

Total gross death rate:

Nosocomial infection rate for each service:

Nosocomial infection rate for the semiannual period:

Postoperative Infection Rate

Another specific type of infection of great concern to hospitals is the **postoperative infection rate.** This is because a postoperative infection can contribute to the increased morbidity, mortality, and cost of care. Postoperative infections occur, as the name suggests, after surgery. Even though hospitals take care to avoid an infection after surgery, one still can occur.

Two terms need to be considered here:

- A *surgical procedure* is defined as any single, separate, systematic process upon or within the body that can be complete in itself; normally is performed by a physician, dentist, or other licensed practitioner; can be performed with or without instruments; and is performed to restore disunited or deficient parts, remove diseased or injured tissues, extract foreign matter, assist in obstetrical delivery, or aid in diagnosis.

- A *surgical operation* is defined as one or more surgical procedures performed at one time for one patient via a common approach or for a common purpose.

  — An example of a surgical operation including more than one surgical procedure is an abdominoperitoneal resection, which involves resection of both the abdomen and the peritoneum.

  — An example of two surgical operations and two surgical procedures is a tonsillectomy followed by a circumcision. Even though the procedures were performed at one time for one patient, the approach to each procedure is different and the two procedures are not performed for a common purpose.

The postoperative infection rate is the ratio of all infections in clean surgical cases to the number of surgical operations performed. A general definition of a **clean surgical case** is one in which no infection existed prior to surgery.

The formula for calculating the postoperative infection rate is:

$$\frac{\textit{Total number of infections in clean surgical cases for a period} \times 100}{\textit{Number of surgical operations for the period}}$$

Example: During November, a hospital reported that 758 surgical operations were performed. The infection prevention committee reported one postoperative infection in a clean surgical case. According to the formula, the postoperative infection rate for November is 0.13 percent.

$$\frac{(1 \times 100)}{758} = \frac{100}{758} = 0.1319 = 0.13\%$$

A postoperative infection may be difficult to determine because it is not always evident whether the patient entered the hospital with an infection or acquired one because of the surgical techniques used. Therefore, the medical staff should provide guidance to the HIM practitioner and the Infection Prevention Department on what constitutes a clean surgical case and which infections should be considered postoperative infections.

Many Infection Prevention Departments use the classifications developed by the National Nosocomial Infections Surveillance System (now a part of the NHSN). These are developed according to the likelihood and degree of wound contamination at the time of the operation. Wounds are classified as clean, clean-contaminated, contaminated, and dirty or infected wounds.

Their descriptions include a clean wound as one in which no inflammation is encountered and the respiratory, alimentary, genital, or uninfected urinary tracts are not entered. Many Infection Prevention Departments report the number of postoperative infections relative to the type of surgery that was performed. For example, if a patient has no infection prior to a coronary artery bypass graft, but develops one after surgery, then the Infection Prevention Department would report this as a postoperative infection in a clean case.

A clean-contaminated case is one in which the respiratory, alimentary, genital, or urinary tract is entered. Specifically, operations involving the biliary tract, appendix, vagina, and oropharynx are included in this category. For instance, a patient who develops an infection after an abdominal hysterectomy would be reported as an infection in a clean-contaminated case.

A contaminated wound includes an open, fresh, accidental wound; an operation with a break in sterile technique or gross spillage from the gastrointestinal tract; and incisions in which acute, nonpurulent inflammation is encountered.

A dirty wound is one that involves existing clinical infection or perforated viscera.

If you are assisting the Infection Prevention Department with their statistics, be sure to determine how they are classifying your facility's postoperative infections.

Exercise 8.3

Based on the information in the table below, calculate (round to two decimal places) the postoperative infection and postoperative death rates for University Hospital during this semiannual period.

University Hospital
Surgery Service
July–December 20XX

Number of surgical operations	2,059
Number of patients operated on	2,053
Number of postoperative infections	12
Number of postoperative deaths	10

Answers:

Postoperative infection rate:

Postoperative death rate:

Exercise 8.4

Based on the information in the table below, calculate (round to two decimal places) the rates requested.

University Hospital
Surgery Service
July–December 20XX Statistics

Month	Dis*	Deaths		Infections		No. of Patients Operated	No. of Surgical Operations
		Postop	Other	Postop	Nosocomial		
Jul	620	3	12	3	5	301	302
Aug	560	2	10	2	4	293	299
Sep	600	2	9	3	3	312	315
Oct	558	4	11	3	4	299	302
Nov	690	3	14	2	3	306	306
Dec	682	4	14	3	2	314	316
Total							

*Deaths are included.

Answers:

1. The month with the lowest postoperative infection rate:

2. The postoperative infection rate for the semiannual period:

3. The month with the highest postoperative death rate:

4. The postoperative death rate for the semiannual period:

5. The gross death rate for the surgical service during the semiannual period:

Complication Rate

In addition to infections, healthcare facilities are concerned with any other type of complication that results from, or occurs during, the course of care. A **complication** is a medical condition that arises during an inpatient hospitalization. According to the Centers for Medicare and Medicaid Services, a complication is a condition that occurs during the patient's hospital stay that extends the length of stay by at least one day in 75 percent of cases.

Complications may be related to the quality of care received by patients. The purpose of collecting complication rates is to determine if changes in the treatment or practice in the facility can prevent them from occurring again.

Examples of complications include blood transfusion reactions, injuries sustained during cardiopulmonary resuscitation, reactions to medications given, vaccination reactions, and patient falls out of bed, just to name a few. Infections, of course, can be complications, but they are generally calculated separately. Any of these examples would change the way the patient was treated from the original reason for hospitalization.

Many facilities calculate these rates at usual intervals: monthly, quarterly, semiannually, or annually.

The general formula for calculating the complication rate is:

$$\frac{Total\ number\ of\ complications\ for\ a\ period \times 100}{Total\ number\ of\ discharges\ in\ the\ period}$$

Example: From January through June, Community Hospital had 14 complications and 1,862 discharges. The complication rate is

$$\frac{(14 \times 100)}{1,862} = 0.75\%$$

More often than not, facilities will calculate specific types of complications.

Example: In August, Community Hospital had 12 patients on the Medicine unit who had a blood transfusion. Of those, two developed an adverse reaction to the transfusion. The blood transfusion reaction rate is calculated by placing the number of blood transfusion reactions (2) × 100 in the numerator and dividing it by the number of blood transfusions.

$$\frac{(2 \times 100)}{12} = 16.67\%$$

Exercise 8.5

Based on the information in the table below for Community Hospital, calculate (round to two decimal places) the complication rate for each service and the total for this semiannual period.

Community Hospital
Statistics
July–December 20XX

Service	Discharges	Complications	Complication Rate
Medicine	1,742	142	
Surgery	1,080	180	
Obstetrics	389	3	
Newborn	390	1	
Total			

Cesarean-Section Rate

Most hospitals determine the percentage of deliveries that are performed by Cesarean section (commonly called C-section) as compared to spontaneous or vaginal deliveries. Much attention has been given to high C-section rates by specific physicians, hospitals, and areas of the country because of concerns about adverse effects to the mother and child. Additionally, it may be necessary to report C-section rates to accrediting agencies or the American Medical Association (AMA) for such reasons as residency programs.

A **delivery** is defined as the process of delivering a live-born infant or dead fetus (and placenta) by manual, instrumental, or surgical means.

> **Handy Tip:** A pregnant mother who delivers has one delivery but may have multiple births. For example, a woman who delivers a live-born infant is counted as one delivery and one live birth whereas a woman who delivers live-born twins is counted as one delivery and two live births. A woman who delivers a stillbirth is counted as one delivery and one intermediate or late fetal death. This is also considered to be one delivery and one birth since a stillbirth is considered to be a birth, but not a live birth.

> **Handy Tip:** Sometimes a woman is admitted to the hospital for a condition of her pregnancy but does not deliver her infant during that hospitalization. For example, a woman may be admitted in apparent labor, which turns out to be false labor. In this case, the patient may be classified as an obstetrics patient, not delivered.

The formula for calculating the Cesarean-section rate is:

$$\frac{\textit{Total number of C-sections performed in a period} \times 100}{\textit{Total number of deliveries in the period (including C-sections)}}$$

Handy Tip: The C-section rate is not based on the number of patients discharged but, rather, on the number of deliveries. A rate compares the number of actual occurrences with the total possible; obviously, only deliveries can be C-sections. Usually the data on deliveries and the number of C-sections for the period are obtained from delivery room personnel.

Example: Three C-sections were performed in a month during which there were 360 deliveries. The C-section rate is calculated by multiplying the number of C-sections (3) by 100 and then dividing that number by the total number of deliveries (360). The C-section rate is 0.83 percent.

$$\frac{(3 \times 100)}{360} = \frac{300}{360} = 0.83\%$$

Exercise 8.6

Based on the information in the table below, calculate (round to two decimal places) the C-section rate and the vaginal delivery rate at University Hospital for the semiannual period.

University Hospital
Obstetrics Service
Semiannual Statistics
January–June 20XX

Admissions	526
Discharges:	
Delivered	394
Not delivered	120
Aborted	12
Vaginal deliveries	316
C-sections	78

Answers:

C-section rate:

Vaginal delivery rate:

Exercise 8.7

Based on the information in the table below, calculate (round to two decimal places) the C-section rate, the newborn death rate, and the fetal death rate at University Hospital for the month of May.

University Hospital
Newborn Service
May 20XX

Discharges (includes deaths)	150
Births:	
Single live births	138
Multiple live births	1 set of twins
	1 set of triplets
Deliveries:	
Vaginal	119
C-section	27
Deaths:	
Newborn	1
Fetal:	
Early	4
Intermediate	3
Late	3

Answers:

C-section rate:

Newborn death rate:

Fetal death rate:

Consultation Rates

A **consultation** is the response by one healthcare professional to another healthcare professional's request to provide recommendations or opinions regarding the care of a particular patient or resident. A patient's attending physician may occasionally request that a consultant (another physician or healthcare practitioner) examine a patient and give an opinion as to his or her condition. Ordinarily the consultant is called in to help identify and treat a patient whose diagnosis is outside the expertise of the attending physician. Consultants are usually specialists in their particular field of medicine. The consultant has the opportunity to visit with the patient and review the medical record and then prepare a consultation report that includes the findings of the examination and recommendations for treating the patient.

The formula for calculating the **consultation rate** is:

$$\frac{Total\ number\ of\ patients\ receiving\ a\ consultation \times 100}{Total\ number\ of\ patients\ discharged}$$

Example: During the past month, a medicine unit had 93 discharges, 12 of whom were seen by a consultant. The consultation rate is 12.9 percent.

$$\frac{(12 \times 100)}{93} = \frac{1,200}{93} = 12.90\%$$

Handy Tip: Close examination of this formula reveals that the definition of a rate applies here. That is, every patient discharged could theoretically have had a consultation.

Exercise 8.8

Based on the information in the table below, calculate the consultation rate (round to two decimal places) at Community Hospital for each service and the total for the semiannual period.

**Community Hospital
Semiannual Statistics
January–June 20XX**

Service	Discharges	No. of Patients Receiving Consultations	Consultation Rate
Medicine	2,880	864	
Surgery	2,160	701	
Obstetrics	685	26	
Psychiatric	142	6	
Rehabilitation	156	12	
Pediatrics	251	42	
Newborn	672	2	
Total			

Exercise 8.9

Based on the information in the table below, calculate (round to two decimal places) the rates requested below for Community Hospital. In this exercise, the deaths are included in the discharges.

Community Hospital
Surgery Service
Annual Statistics 20XX

Month	Discharges	Deaths	Consultations	Consultation Rate	Gross Death Rate
January	576	17	115		
February	589	12	102		
March	601	15	84		
April	542	13	63		
May	614	6	96		
June	574	14	85		
July	563	10	74		
August	555	9	69		
September	603	6	78		
October	591	7	45		
November	583	5	86		
December	562	12	73		
Total					

1. Consultation rate for each month:

2. Consultation rate for the year for the surgery service:

3. Gross death rate for each month:

4. Gross death rate for the year for the surgery service:

Other Rates

The HIM practitioner may compute and report other rates according to individual healthcare facility needs. External agencies may also ask that additional data and rates be reported. To pursue all the possibilities in this book is impractical. The best rule of thumb is to use the "other rates" formula. You may become so intrigued with this formula that you will volunteer to produce new and useful rates, which is, incidentally, part of the HIM professional's responsibility. The formula for calculating other rates is:

$$\frac{Number\ of\ times\ something\ happened \times 100}{Number\ of\ times\ something\ could\ have\ happened}$$

Handy Tip: Statistics should not be kept just because they have always been kept. After you assure yourself, the administration, and the medical staff that a particular statistic no longer serves a useful purpose, stop keeping it. Do not be afraid to be creative and imaginative about providing new ideas for statistical computations that will serve a useful purpose, even if only on a temporary, special-study basis.

Exercise 8.10

Based on the information in the table below, calculate (round to two decimal places) the readmission rates requested below for University Hospital, using the following formula:

$$\frac{Number\ of\ patients\ readmitted\ within\ 30\ days\ of\ the\ previous\ discharge \times 100}{Total\ patients\ discharged\ (including\ deaths)}$$

University Hospital
Surgery Service
Semiannual Statistics
January–June 20XX

Month	No. Of Patients Discharged Alive	No. of Patients Readmitted within 30 Days of the Previous Discharge	Readmission Rate
January	562	27	
February	654	32	
March	678	38	
April	649	21	
May	658	25	
June	667	34	
Total			

1. The readmission rate for each month:

2. The total readmission rate for the period:

Exercise 8.11

Using the information below, for the next two exercises calculate the readmission rates for Community Medical Center and Community Meadows Medical Center. Express in a percent. (Round to two decimal places.)

Community Medical Center
Annual Statistics, 20XX

Discharges (Includes Deaths)	Deaths	No. of Patients Readmitted	Readmission Rate
9,305	440	903	

Community Meadows Medical Center
Annual Statistics, 20XX

Discharges (Includes Deaths)	Deaths	No. of Patients Readmitted	Readmission Rate
8,870	501	672	

Exercise 8.12

Based on the information in the table below, calculate (round to two decimal places) the rate of nondelivered patients and aborted patients at University Hospital for each month and for the quarter.

University Hospital
Obstetrics Department
Fourth Quarter Statistics, 20XX

Month	No. of Patients Delivered	No. of Patients Not Delivered	No. of Patients Aborted	Nondelivered Rate	Abortion Rate
October	402	12	6		
November	385	20	5		
December	391	18	3		
Total					

Exercise 8.13

Based on the information in the table below for University Hospital, calculate (round to two decimal places) the rate of accounts turned over to collection for each month and for the period. Use the formula for a rate to make these calculations.

**University Hospital
Semiannual Statistics
July–December 20XX**

Month	No. of Discharges	No. of Accounts Turned Over to a Collection Agency	Rate of Accounts Turned Over to a Collection Agency
July	302	25	
August	326	30	
September	342	32	
October	318	15	
November	352	24	
December	312	19	
Total			

Exercise 8.14

Based on the information in the table below, calculate (round to two decimal places) the rates requested.

**Community Hospital
Medicine Service
Selected Annual Statistics, 20XX**

Total Hospital Discharges: 7,201

Medicine Service	Number
Discharges	4,523
Complications	125
Nosocomial infections	78
Deaths (included in discharges)	60
Payer information:	
Medicare	905
Medicaid	812
Third-party insurance	2,126
Self-pay	680

(continued on next page)

Exercise 8.14 (continued)

Selected patients:

Primary diagnosis:

Cancer	986
Diabetes and its complications	625
HIV/AIDS	123
Myocardial infarction	450
Asthma	267
Substance abuse	98

Answers:

Percentage of total hospital patients in the Medicine service:

Complication rate in the Medicine service:

Nosocomial infection rate in the Medicine service:

Gross death rate in the Medicine service:

Percentage of patients with:
Medicare:

Medicaid:

Third-party insurance:

Self-pay:

Exercise 8.14 (continued)

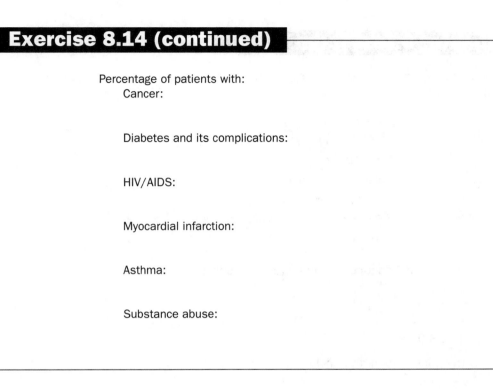

Percentage of patients with:
Cancer:

Diabetes and its complications:

HIV/AIDS:

Myocardial infarction:

Asthma:

Substance abuse:

Chapter 8 Test

Indicate whether the following statements are true or false.

1. Every healthcare facility must keep infection rates for each of its medical care units.

2. A nosocomial infection is an infection that was acquired while a patient was hospitalized.

3. The postoperative infection rate is the ratio of all infections in clean surgical cases to the number of surgical procedures.

4. A patient who has a salpingo-oophorectomy would be counted as having one surgical procedure and one surgical operation.

5. A patient who had a colonoscopy and removal of two moles on his neck at the same time would be counted as having one surgical operation and two procedures.

(continued on next page)

Chapter 8 Test (continued)

Complete statements 6 and 7 using the annual statistics reported in the table below.

Discharges:	
Adults and children	7,280
Newborn	798
Surgical procedures	1,265
Surgical operations	1,260
Patients receiving consultations	1,999
Nosocomial infections	23

6. The hospital acquired infection rate (including newborns) is:

    a. 0.02%

    b. 0.28%

    c. 2.80%

    d. 28.00%

7. The consultation rate (including newborns) is:

    a. 0.02%

    b. 0.24%

    c. 2.75%

    d. 24.75%

8. A hospital reports the following statistics for the past year: births, 1,345; deliveries, 1,340; C-sections, 60; and obstetrical discharges, 1,425. The C-section rate for that year is:

    a. 0.47%

    b. 1.47%

    c. 4.48%

    d. 44.78%

9. A women's hospital reported 212 deliveries during June. Two sets of twins were born. There were 215 obstetrical discharges and 214 births; four women had first-time C-sections and three women had a repeat C-section. The C-section rate for June is 3.30 percent. True or false?

10. What is the percentage of multiple births?

    a. 0.93%

    b. 93.5%

    c. 1.87%

    d. 0.94%

Chapter 8 Test (continued)

11. What is the percentage of patients with multiple births?

    a. 0.93%
    b. 0.94%
    c. 94.0%
    d. 0.65%

12. A third-party review company reported the statistics in the table below. Calculate (round to two decimal places) the rate of admissions approved for each month and for the quarter.

	July	August	September
Number of admission claims reviewed	927	935	956
Number of claims approved for admission to the hospital	912	927	931

Answers:

July:

August:

September:

Quarter:

Chapter 9
Statistics Computed within the Health Information Management Department

Key Terms

Budget

Capital budget

Case-mix index

Electronic health record

Electronic signature

Fiscal year

Full-time equivalent employee

Hybrid health record

Operational budget

Payback period

Productivity

Profiling

Return on investment

Spreadsheet

Unit labor cost

Objectives

At the conclusion of this chapter, you should be able to:

- Describe the uses of statistics computed within the HIM department in terms of unit cost, productivity, and staffing levels

- Recognize how statistics are used in the creation of the health information department budget

- Define budget and differentiate between the operational and capital budgets

- Verify computerized statistical reports for accuracy

- Recalculate statistics for greater specificity

- Generate computerized statistical reports

Health Information Statistics

Statistics computed for use within the health information management (HIM) department usually relate to labor costs, productivity, and staffing, and often are used in determining whether the department may be able to hire a new employee, set benchmarks for productivity, determine absentee rates, and so on. The following sections provide examples of common, everyday computations made by HIM staff members.

Employee Compensation and Unit Labor Costs

One example of where health information managers must make effective decisions is in regard to employee compensation and **unit labor cost.**

The annual compensation for an individual employee is calculated by multiplying the number of hours worked per year (2,080 for a full-time employee) by the hourly wage and then multiplying that number by the benefits received. A sample calculation would be:

2,080 hours × $10 per hour × 30% benefits = $20,800 × .30 = $6,240 + $20,800 = $27,040

> **Handy Tip:** A quicker way to compute this is to multiply by 1.3 (if 30% benefits).
>
> 2,080 hours × $10 per hour × 1.3 (30% benefits) = $27,040

To determine the annual productivity, multiply the amount of work completed (for example, lines transcribed, number of records coded and the like) per day by the number of workdays in the year (5 workdays per week × 52 weeks per year = 260 workdays). Note that this calculation includes any vacation time or sick leave that an employee may take.

The unit labor cost is determined by dividing the total annual compensation by total annual productivity. For example, workload in a transcription section of a department is commonly measured in lines or minutes of dictation transcribed by the staff. To determine the unit transcription labor cost, divide the total transcriptionist annual compensation by the total annual productivity as shown below.

$$\frac{Total\ (sum)\ medical\ transcriptionist\ annual\ compensation}{Total\ (sum)\ medical\ transcriptionist\ annual\ productivity}$$

Example: Two full-time beginning transcriptionists in the HIM department produce 1,000 lines each per day. One employee earns $12.00 per hour and is paid an annual salary of $24,960; the other employee earns $15.00 per hour and is paid an annual salary of $31,200.

To determine the annual productivity, multiply the number of lines transcribed by the two employees (1,000 per day per transcriptionist or 2,000 per day) by the number of workdays in the year (5 workdays per week × 52 weeks per year = 260 workdays).

2(260 workdays × 1,000 lines) = 520,000 lines per year

To determine the unit cost, add the two salaries ($24,960 + $31,200 = $56,160) and divide by the total number of lines transcribed by the two employees in one year (520,000). The unit cost is $0.108 or 11 cents per line.

$$\frac{\$56,160}{520,000} = \$0.108 = \$0.11$$

Example: This formula can be applied to other employees in the department. For example, one coder is compensated at $12.00 per hour and codes six records per hour. The employee's annual compensation is $24,960.

To determine the employee's annual productivity, multiply six records per hour by 7.5 hours per day to get 45 records per day. Then multiply 45 by 5 days in the workweek and 52 weeks in the year to get 11,700 records coded per year. The unit cost is $2.13 per record.

Handy Tip: Some employers consider 7.5 hours a productive work day, thinking in terms of an 8-hour day minus breaks the employee may take.

Handy Tip: Notice that the unit cost did not consider times that the employee is not working (for example, sick time or vacation time). The unit cost to code one record is still valid because someone has to perform the work even when the employee who normally performs that task is absent.

Exercise 9.1

Complete the exercises below.

1. Transcriptionist A is a full-time employee earning $13.00 per hour and an annual salary of $27,040. She transcribes 1,200 lines per day for a total of 312,000 lines per year. What is the unit medical transcription labor cost for transcriptionist A (or, how much does a line cost when transcribed by transcriptionist A)?

2. Transcriptionist B is a full-time employee earning $12.00 per hour and an annual salary of $24,960. He transcribes 900 lines per day for a total of 234,000 lines per year. What is the unit medical transcription labor cost for transcriptionist B?

3. A HIM department has eight full-time transcriptionists. Five of them produce 1,000 lines each per day. Of these five, one earns $12.00 per hour, three earn $12.50 per hour, and one earns $15.00 per hour.

   Two other transcriptionists in the department produce 1,100 lines per day. Of these two, one earns $13.00 per hour and the other earns $16.00 per hour. Finally, the eighth transcriptionist produces 1,200 lines per day and earns $12.00 per hour.

   a. What is the difference in cost per line between the employee who produces 1,000 lines per day and makes $12.00 per hour and the employee who produces 1,200 lines per day and makes $12.00 per hour?
   b. What general observations can you make about the unit labor cost and the two employees just mentioned?
   c. What is the difference in cost per line between the employee who produces 1,000 lines per day and makes $15.00 per hour and the employee who produces 1,100 lines per day and makes $13.00 per hour?
   d. What is the total unit cost for medical transcription?

To justify costs for releases of information (ROI) in the health information department, one HIM professional needed to calculate cost breakdowns. (See table 9.1.)

The Health Insurance Portability and Accountability Act (HIPAA), commonly referred to as the Privacy Rule, allows a facility to charge a reasonable, cost-based fee for any requests for records made by patients after the first request. The first request each year must be made without charge to the patient. Time studies would need to be performed in order to validate the cost. This may involve:

- Keeping track of the time it takes to review the request and log it into your computer system

- Finding the patient information in the master patient index

- Determining the location of the medical record, either paper or electronic

- Determining whether other departments have portions of the medical record and have possibly made a disclosure

- Retrieving the record if it is a paper record or locating the record online and printing any scanned documents

- Reviewing any previous disclosures made

Table 9.1.   Average record requests per month

Community Hospital Health Information Department Release of Information Costs Average Requests per Month = 360	
Item	**Cost per Request**
Postage: $305 per month	$\dfrac{\$305}{360} = 0.847 = \$0.85$
Service contract (includes copier): $100 per month	$\dfrac{\$100}{360} = 0.277 = \$0.28$
Equipment (includes copies): $125 per month	$\dfrac{\$125}{360} = 0.347 = \$0.35$
Supplies (includes toner, printer cartridges, paper): $75 per month	$\dfrac{\$75}{360} = 0.208 = \$0.21$
Wages: $12.00 per hour = monthly salary of $2,080 ($12.00 × 2,080 hours = $24,960; $\dfrac{\$24,960}{12} = \$2,080$)	$\dfrac{\$2,080}{360} = 5.777 = \$5.78$
Total	**$7.47**

- Preparing a list of the disclosures

- Preparing an invoice for the patient

- Updating the release of the information log

The HIM department also may consider nonlabor expenses such as those listed in table 9.1. However, the facility's chief financial officer is usually consulted to determine whether other nonlabor costs can be applied.

Another aspect that will need consideration is that some health information departments are copying records onto a CD or compact disc and giving them directly to a patient. This will affect the cost of the release of information as it does not take as much time to copy the parts of the record onto a CD or thumb drive as it would to produce a paper copy. Also, when Health Information Exchanges become fully operational, it may be possible to move the information from one organization to another. The Health Information Director will need to calculate the time needed to transfer the information rather than copy the information.

Exercise 9.2

Using the information in the table below, calculate the cost breakdown per item and the monthly cost for the release of information (ROI) services at Community Hospital.

Community Hospital
Health Information Department
Release of Information Costs
Average Requests per Month = 482

Item	Cost per Month
Postage	$365
Service contract (includes copier)	$85
Equipment (includes copies)	$122
Supplies (includes toner, printer cartridges, paper)	$92
Wages	$12.50 per hour
Monthly cost	

Exercise 9.3

Using the information provided in the table below, complete the following exercises.

Community Hospital
Health Information Department
Release of Information Costs
Average Requests per Month = 542

Item	Cost per Month
Postage	$456
Service contract (includes copier)	$216
Equipment (includes copies)	$135
Supplies (includes toner, printer cartridges, paper)	$110
Wages	$13.00 per hour

1. Calculate the cost breakdown for each item.

2. What is the monthly cost for the ROI services?

3. On average, the ROI section brings in $1,800 per month. What is the difference between cost and income?

Other Labor Unit Costs

The HIM department also processes patient record (chart) requests, which consumes a great deal of staff time. Responsibilities in maintaining records include:

- *Chart pulls*: Even as the need to pull records of previous patients diminishes with the use of an **electronic health record** (EHR), the HIM department will still need to determine costs and productivity standards for this work. A combination of paper and electronic records will continue to be in use for some time, and both manual and electronic processes will be used to maintain the record. This combination is referred to as a **hybrid health record.** The types of statistics may include the number of requests for the paper record versus electronic records or the number needed as stat (immediately) versus routine requests.

- *Scanning of records*: Some facilities choose to scan the paper record to make it available online. These facilities may have an electronic document management system (EDMS) to help manage all their documents for a patient. This new technology allows users to scan documents, move documents from the transcription system to the EHR, enter information online, handle the **electronic signature** of records, index documents as they are entered into the computer system, and access information from a variety of locations, to name a few functions. This will determine the types of statistics needed to assess who is using the system, how the electronic signature is given, where providers are signing, and so forth. New technologies will continue to evolve, and managers in health information departments will continue to determine the costs and benefits of these new systems.

- *Provider–patient e-mail*: As patients become more comfortable with e-mailing their physicians and as healthcare insurers begin to reimburse physicians for their time used to e-mail patients, this will become an everyday issue for healthcare organizations. E-mail and text messages are considered to be healthcare business records and thus are subject to the same rules and regulations as any other health record. E-mail can be used to schedule appointments, refill prescriptions, or transfer department results. Organizations may decide to keep track of the time spent responding to e-mails, gathering information before the e-mail is answered, and deciding what can be answered via e-mail.

- *Loose papers*: The number of pieces of paper received in the HIM department for filing is a significant factor in determining staffing levels. Loose papers may be measured in inches or by individual pieces, which is a more accurate measure. Because of the time involved in tracking this information, departments may choose to sample this activity for a one-week period several times a year.

Exercise 9.4

Complete the following two exercises.

1. The HIM department at Community Hospital completed a time study, and the data are listed in the table below. Complete the table by determining the number of hours worked in each activity.

Community Hospital
Health Information Department
Time Allocation Report
September 20XX

Service/Division	Number of Hours	Hours Worked
Inpatient records:		
Pediatrics	11.75 h/w x 4 weeks	
Obstetrics	59.5 h/w x 4 weeks	
Psychiatric	98.5 h/w x 4 weeks	
Newborn	50.75 h/w x 4 weeks	
Medicine	426.75 h/w x 4 weeks	
Surgery	447 h/w x 4 weeks	
Subtotal inpatient records		
ED records:		
Clerical/Processing	28 h/w x 4 weeks	
Correspondence	7 h/w x 4 weeks	
Supervisory	5 h/w x 4 weeks	
Subtotal ED records		
General clinic:		
Clerical/Processing	6 h/w x 4 weeks	
Supervisory	0.5 h/w x 4 weeks	
Transcription	0.10 h/record x 170 records	
Subtotal general clinic		

Exercise 9.4 (continued)

Outpatient/Ambulatory surgery

Clerical/Primary:	21.5 h/w x 4 weeks
Filing	5.25 h/w x 4 weeks
Admissions	2.5 h/w x 4 weeks
Combining records	1 h/w x 4 weeks
Tumor registry	1 h/w x 4 weeks
Correspondence	0.25 h/w x 4 weeks
Record completion	10.75 h/w x 4 weeks
Certificates	3.25 h/w x 4 weeks
Supervisory	5 h/w x 4 weeks
Transcription	0.10 h/record x 620 records
Coding	0.12 h/record x 850 records

**Subtotal outpatient/
Ambulatory surgery**

Total hours worked

2. What percentage of the total hours is spent in each category of inpatient records, and what percentage is spent in inpatient, emergency department, general clinical, and outpatient/ambulatory surgery records? Round to two decimal places.

Service/Area	% of Time Worked
Pediatrics	
Obstetrics	
Psychiatric	
Newborn	
Medicine	
Surgery	
All inpatient records	
ED records	
General clinic records	
Outpatient/Ambulatory surgery records	

Exercise 9.5

Your physician clinic's chief financial officer has determined that it costs the clinic $3.75 per telephone call for the receptionist to set up an appointment with a physician in the clinic compared to $1.50 per online request to set up an appointment. What would the per appointment cost savings be if, during one day at the clinic, 150 patient appointments were arranged by online request rather than by telephone?

Exercise 9.6

1. The Health Information Committee has requested information about the electronic signature system being used in your facility. They would like to know the locations where physicians are accessing the system. Review the information in the table below and determine the percentage of use from each site. Round to one decimal place.

Community Hospital
Electronic Signature System
250 Physicians on Staff; 231 Using the System

Site	No. of Physicians Using the System at This Site	% of Physicians Using the System at This Site
Medicine, 2 West	45	
Medicine, 2 East	35	
Pediatrics, 3 West	20	
Obstetrics, 1 West	9	
Physician's lounge	65	
HIM department	42	
Personal mobile device	5	
Physician home	15	

2. What is the percentage of physicians not using the electronic signature system? Round to one decimal place.

Exercise 9.7

Loose sheets continue to come to the HIM department even after the implementation of a hybrid electronic health record. Using the data provided in the table, compute the data requested below.

**Community Hospital
Health Information Services
Loose Sheet Report
July 20XX**

Department	Week #1	Week #2	Week #3	Week #4	Total	Proportion
Lab	27	34	48	54		
Radiology	15	21	26	42		
Pathology	25	26	28	31		
Nursing	17	22	36	41		
Physical therapy	5	4	2	12		
Miscellaneous	20	21	22	26		
Total						

1. The totals for each department and each week:

2. The proportion of loose sheets received from each department:

Productivity

Productivity is defined as a unit of performance defined by management in quantitative standards. Productivity allows organizations to measure how well the organization converts input into output, or labor into a product or service.

Most HIM departments have productivity standards for different areas in the department. For example, in the coding section, a productivity standard may be that employees should code four inpatient records per hour. In a 7.5-hour workday (taking into account breaks the employee will take), 30 inpatient records would be coded per day. But how does the HIM manager or supervisor know how many records should be coded in a day? A number of factors influence this decision. Some things the supervisor should consider are:

- Does the coder do anything in addition to coding, such as abstracting, answering the phone, or obtaining additional information about the diagnoses and procedures?

- What kinds of records is the coder coding? Are they long lengths of stay or short? Are they complex cases or relatively simple cases to code?

In their article in the *Journal of AHIMA,* P. J. Miller and F. Waterstraat suggested two simple formulas that accurately calculate labor productivity (Miller and Waterstraat 2004):

$$Completed\ work = Total\ work\ output - Defective\ work$$

and

$$Labor\ productivity = \frac{Completed\ work}{Hours\ worked\ to\ produce\ total\ work\ output}$$

Determining the total work output and the hours worked is clear; however, determining the defective work involves auditing the work to determine if any work is defective. Miller and Waterstraat describe three ways to audit employees' work output. First, the manager could perform a review of all the work performed; second, the manager could perform a review of work chosen through a random sample; or third, the manager could use a fixed-percent random sample audit. The last suggestion is the easiest. This method requires the manager to select a fixed percent of an employee's total work for review. The manager also has a predetermined quality standard in mind and then reviews the work and classifies it as completed work or defective work. Additional work could be reviewed if more information is needed to determine the type of defect or until all the work has been reviewed.

Table 9.2 shows the calculation for determining inpatient coding productivity for one month.

Notice in table 9.2 that Coder D's average work output is 4.69 records per hour ($\frac{work\ output}{total\ hours\ worked} = \frac{375}{80} = 4.69$). However, after auditing the work, it was determined that 240 of those records were coded accurately (completed work output). Coder D's completed work is really 3.00 ($\frac{240}{80} = 3.00$).

Staffing Levels

Healthcare organizations use a variety of methods to determine appropriate staffing levels. For example, many outpatient facilities use patient encounters per **full-time equivalent employee** (FTE) per month. A patient encounter is any personal contact between a patient and a physician or other person authorized to furnish healthcare services for the diagnosis or treatment of the patient. These may include laboratory services, x-ray services, physical therapy, and other ancillary services.

The staffing level is determined by dividing the number of patient encounters by the expected productivity. An FTE is the total number of workers, including part-time, in an area as the equivalent of full-time positions. The number of FTEs does not always equal the actual number of employees because two or more part-time employees might equal one FTE.

$$\frac{Patient\ encounters}{Productivity} = Number\ of\ FTEs\ needed$$

Example: A small physician clinic experiences 300 patient encounters per day. A coder is expected to code 100 records per day. To determine the number of coders needed, divide 300 by 100. Thus, three coders are needed to perform the coding for the physician clinic each day.

Handy Tip: When computing FTE, the manager does not ordinarily round up or down. The reason is that managers must justify the need for any employees. For example, the administration may only want to approve a person working 20% time (0.2 FTE) if a full-time employee is not needed to perform the work.

Table 9.2.   Inpatient coding productivity calculation for one month

Coder	Work Output (All Records Coded)	Total Hours Worked	Average Work Output per Hour	Completed Work Percentage	Completed Work Output (Records Coded Accurately)	Completed Work per Hours Worked
A	500	140	3.57	91%	455	3.25
B	475	140	3.39	96%	456	3.26
C	300	80	3.75	96%	240	3.00
D	375	80	4.69	64%	240	3.00
Department Average			**3.69**			**3.13**

Work Output: number of work units as recorded by the employee or the process

Total Hours Worked: number of hours worked by the employee to produce work, which does not include time for meals, breaks, and meetings

Average Work Output per Hour: work output divided by total hours worked

Completed Work Percentage: percentage of completed work from audit

Completed Work Output: work output multiplied by completed work percentage

Completed Work per Hours Worked: completed work output divided by total hours worked

Hospital HIM departments often use discharges as their method to determine staff levels.

Example: To determine the number of employees needed in a coding section, the health information manager first multiplies the average number of inpatient records coded per hour (6) by the number of hours in the workday (7.5), which amounts to 45 records coded per day. Hospital discharges numbered approximately 55 inpatients per day. Based on this number, the manager then calculated that she needed 1.2 FTEs to accomplish the coding task.

$$\frac{55}{45} = 1.2 \text{ FTE}$$

In this example, the manager would need one full-time employee plus one 0.2 FTE, which is computed as 40 hours per week multiplied by 0.2. Thus, she would need another employee to work eight hours per week to handle the workload.

Here's another way to determine the number of employees needed. Determine how many minutes and hours it would take to perform all the work then divide by the number of productive hours. For example, an HIM Director would like to know how many FTEs are needed to analyze the weekly discharges in her facility. There are 350 discharges per week. It takes one employee 15 minutes to analyze one record. Using a productive week as 32 hours, the Director determines that she will need 2.7 employees to analyze the week's discharges.

$$15 \text{ minutes} \times 350 \text{ records} = 5,250 \text{ minutes}$$

$$\frac{5,250 \text{ minutes}}{60 \text{ minutes (in one hour)}} = 87.5 \text{ hours}$$

$$\frac{87.5 \text{ hours}}{32 \text{ productive hours}} = 2.7 \text{ FTE}$$

Exercise 9.8

1. Community Physician's Clinic is a large clinic with 85 physicians. They treat about 8,600 patients each week. Coders are expected to code 100 clinic records each day. How many FTEs are needed to code these records? (Assume a five-day work week.)

2. Community Physician's Clinic is buying the Medical Center Physician's Clinic. They will be adding 24 physicians who treat 62,400 patients per year. There are no credentialed coders employed at Medical Center Physician's Clinic. The Coding Supervisor at Community Physician's Clinic will be responsible for adding coders to her current staff. The coders will be expected to code 100 clinical records per day. How many more FTEs will be needed to code these records?

Exercise 9.9

1. Community Hospital wants to make the transition to an electronic data management system. The process will involve scanning 5,000 inpatient records, 2,000 outpatient records, and 1,000 ED records into the new system. The hospital estimates that there are 30 pages per inpatient record, 4 pages per outpatient record, and 4 pages per ED record. Assuming that one scanning clerk can scan 1,500 pages per day, how many days will it take to complete the transition?

2. Use the scenario in the question above to answer this question: The HIM Department would like to complete this project in 30 days. How many FTEs will the HIM Department manager need to hire to complete this in a month?

3. Use the information in the table below to answer the following questions. Each employee worked eight-hour days during the 21 workdays in September. Round all answers to two decimal places.

   a. What percentage of the total number of records did each employee code during the month?
   b. How many records is each coder coding each workday?
   c. How many records is each coder coding per hour? (Use an eight-hour workday.)
   d. How many minutes does it take each coder to code one record?
   e. What percentage of records is not passing the quality screens for each coder?

Community Hospital
Health Information Management Department
Coding Section—Productive and Quality Audit Reports
September 20XX

Coder	No. of Records Coded	No. of Records Not Passing Quality Screens
A	425	4
B	502	3
C	373	11

Exercise 9.9 (continued)

Answers:

a. What percentage of the total number of records did each employee code during the month?

Coder A:

Coder B:

Coder C:

b. How many records is each coder coding each workday?

Coder A:

Coder B:

Coder C:

c. How many records is each coder coding per hour?

Coder A:

Coder B:

Coder C:

d. On average, how many minutes does it take each coder to code one record?

Coder A:

Coder B:

Coder C:

(continued on next page)

Exercise 9.9 (continued)

e. What percentage of records is not passing the quality screens for each coder?

Coder A:

Coder B:

Coder C:

Exercise 9.10

An HIM manager must determine the number of FTEs needed to code 500 discharges per week. It takes 20 minutes to code each record. Each coder works 32 productive hours per week. Round to one digit after the decimal.

How many FTEs will the HIM manager need?

Budgets

If you are responsible for supervising a group of employees, you will most likely also be responsible for budgeting. Usually health information departments are involved with expense and capital budgets.

A **budget** is a plan that converts the organization's goals and objectives into targets for revenue and spending. Planning for the budget begins several months before the facility's **fiscal year** begins. During the planning process, the HIM supervisor uses skills learned in statistics to help approximate the department's expenses for the coming year. Departmental expenses may include employee wages and benefits, supplies, travel and education, membership dues, subscriptions, postage, copying, and equipment maintenance contracts.

The HIM department may also generate some revenue for the department, for example, if it is responsible for the ROI activity or provides a transcription or coding service for the hospital's physicians.

> **Handy Tip:** A fiscal year is a consecutive 12-month period used by an organization as its accounting period. The fiscal year does not have to be a calendar year. For example, the US government's fiscal year begins October 1 and ends September 30. It can be any 12-month period.

Operational Budget

During the year, usually each month, a department director receives budget reports showing amounts budgeted and actual amounts spent. This report generally alerts the department director as to whether or not he or she is over or under budget. Any differences between the budgeted amount and the amount actually spent are called variances. As will be discussed in chapter 10, a variance is a disagreement between two parts. The variance can be used as a device to monitor the department's activities. Budgets also may be available on the organization's Intranet for viewing at any time. This is an easy way for the manager to stay aware of his or her department's budget.

The department director should check the budget report at least each month to determine whether any adjustments must be made in order to stay within the budget. Often the director may be required to explain why the department is over or under budget. This assessment of a department's financial transactions to identify differences between the budget amount and the actual amount of a line item is called a variance analysis.

To determine the variance, subtract the budgeted amount from the actual amount and then divide the difference by the budgeted amount.

Item	Budget	Actual	Variance
Supplies	$3,000	$4,000	($1,000)
Education/training	$1,000	$2,000	($1,000)

Using the information in the preceding table, the variance for supplies is $1,000, or 33.3 percent, over budget.

$$\$4,000 - \$3,000 = \$1,000$$

$$\frac{(\$1,000 \times 100)}{\$3,000} = 33.3\%$$

The variance for education and training is $1,000, or 100 percent, over budget.

$$\$2,000 - \$1,000 = \$1,000$$

$$\frac{(\$1,000 \times 100)}{\$1,000} = 100\%$$

The variances computed above are examples of unfavorable variances, that is, the amounts spent were more than the amounts budgeted.

Favorable variances occur when the amounts actually spent are less than or equal to the amounts budgeted, as shown in the table below.

Item	Budget	Actual	Variance
Supplies	$10,000	$8,000	$2,000
Education/training	$3,500	$2,000	$1,500

In this example, the variance for supplies is $2,000, or 20 percent, under budget.

$$\$10,000 - \$8,000 = \$2,000$$

$$\frac{(\$2,000 \times 100)}{\$10,000} = 20\%$$

The variance for education and training is $1,500, or 42.9 percent, under budget.

$$\$3,500 - \$2,000 = \$1,500$$

$$\frac{(\$1,500 \times 100)}{\$3,500} = 42.9\%$$

Capital Budget

The **capital budget** accounts for the major assets the facility will purchase during the fiscal year, for example, equipment for the HIM department. Capital budget items usually are "high-dollar" purchases. Each facility defines what "high-dollar" means. For example, one facility may consider any assets purchased at a cost of more than $500 to be part of the capital budget.

Moreover, items included in a capital budget usually have a "life" of more than one year; that is, each item's usefulness should last longer than a year. Occasionally, the health information technician (HIT) is involved in assisting the department director in a cost justification for the capital budget. This is very important because only a certain amount of dollars can be allocated to the facility's departments and supervisors wish to have their projects approved. The department director may ask the supervisor to calculate the **payback period** of the project. The payback period provides information on how long it will take the project to recover its costs. The formula is:

$$\frac{Total\ cost\ of\ project}{Annual\ incremental\ cash\ flow}$$

The annual incremental cash flow refers to the savings that a department realizes from the project. For example, if the HIM department needs a new copy machine, the department director may ask the department supervisor to determine, first, how much a new copy machine costs and, then, what kind of savings would be realized from the purchase of a new machine. The supervisor would investigate the cost from different vendors and then calculate an estimate of the savings. Savings considerations might include the time not spent recopying pages, fixing the copy machine, or releasing papers trapped in the machine, as well as the cost of additional paper.

Example: A new copy machine costs $3,000, and the department will realize a savings of $1,000 per year. The payback period is calculated as $\frac{\$3,000}{\$1,000} = 3$ years. There are some disadvantages to using the payback period because it assumes that there will always be the same amount of savings each year. In this example, it is possible that the savings may be less in the second or third year of use due to the aging of the equipment.

Another useful way that department supervisors determine cost justification is by the **return on investment** (ROI). ROI provides information on the rate at which cash is recovered from an investment project. The formula for computing ROI is:

$$\frac{Average\ annual\ incremental\ cash\ flow}{Total\ cost\ of\ the\ project}$$

Using the figures in the example above, the calculation is:

$$\frac{\$1,000 \times 100}{\$3,000} = 33.3\%$$

If 33.3 percent is greater than the facility's required rate of return, the copy machine may be a good investment. Other, more complex formulae are used to determine whether a particular project or major item can be undertaken; however, these formulae are generally performed by the facility's financial department.

Exercise 9.11

Complete the following exercises.

1. In deciding whether to purchase or lease a new dictation system, the HIM supervisor calculates the payback period. The hospital's required payback period is three years. If the equipment costs $28,000 and generates $3,500 per year in savings, what would be the payback period for this equipment? Should the department purchase this equipment?

2. The coding section in the HIM department shows its first-quarter budget analysis as having an expected cost of operation of $62,000. However, the actual cost of operation was $76,000. Calculate the budget variance. Round to one decimal place.

Verification of Statistical Reports

Many statistical reports in healthcare settings are computer-generated. However, a computer can only calculate statistics from the data that are entered. Standardization of terminology, data elements, and formulas from sources such as those found in appendix A will produce data that are more reliable and useful.

When a computerized statistical report is received, the HIM professional should examine it carefully. For example, he or she should verify the total number of discharges listed in a report from coded records and compare it against the total number of discharges according to the census data. Do the totals match? If not, it is important to find out why. Perhaps one of the discharges was not coded. Moreover, computerized statistical reports often give only whole numbers. Thus, the HIM professional may need to calculate certain statistics (for example, death rates) and carry them out to the second decimal place to make the information more valuable to administration or medical staff. Tables or graphs can be created to display a portion of a computerized statistical report. (See chapter 11.)

Computerized Discharge Reports

Figure 9.1 on pages 156 and 157 shows a sample computerized discharge analysis report indicating that the average length of stay (ALOS) of total patients is 7.25 days. To verify this information, use your knowledge of ALOS and recalculate. The calculation is:

$$\frac{4,713}{650} = 7.25$$

Figure 9.1.   Computerized discharge analysis report

* * * YOUR UTILIZATION PROGRAM * * *

	HOSPITAL DAYS									PATIENTS OPERATED	EMERGENCY ADMISSIONS	CONSULTATION	
	TOTAL			AGE ANALYSIS								NO. OF PATIENTS	NUMBER RECEIVED
				0-13 YEARS		14-64 YEARS		65 AND OVER					
SERVICE	PATIENTS	DAYS	AVG. STAY	PAT.	DAYS	PAT.	DAYS	PAT.	DAYS				
1	2	3	4	5	6	7	8	9	10	11	12	13	14
MEDICINE	204	1880	9.2	1	2	161	1300	42	578	170	3	128	209
CARDIOLOGY	60	626	10.4			43	436	17	190	44	1	17	21
ENDOCRINOLOGY	2	23	11.5			2	23			2		2	3
GASTROENTEROL	13	99	7.6			13	99			13		6	11
ONCOLOGY	17	178	10.5			10	112	7	66	16		8	15
PULMONARY MED	4	40	10.0			4	40			4		1	1
PSYCHIATRY	3	17	5.7			2	14	1	3	1		2	6
OB-LIVE BIR	26	114	4.4			26	114			25		2	3
OB-NOT DELIV	9	23	2.6			9	23			4			
OB-ABOR FETUS	15	26	1.7			15	26			15		1	1
GYNECOLOGY	33	125	3.8			33	125			31		5	11
NEWBORN	25	130	5.2	25	130					6			
PED MED	47	265	5.6	44	217	3	48			30	1	8	11
PED SURG	5	11	2.2	4	9	1	2			5		2	2
PED ORTHO	5	27	5.4	2	10	3	17			5		4	5
PED RHINOLARYN	2	3	1.5	1	1	1	2			1		1	1
PED OPHTH	1	2	2.0	1	2					1		1	1
PED UROL	1	1	1.0	1	1					1			
SURGERY	35	222	6.3	1	2	31	190	3	30	34	2	13	18
CV SURG	7	74	10.6			6	72	1	2	7		4	5
ORTHOPEDICS	77	551	7.2	1	11	73	506	3	34	74	1	51	78
PLAS SURG	4	8	2.0			4	8			4		1	1
PROCTOLOGY	1	5	5.0			1	5			1			
ORAL SURG-ADU	3	6	2.0			3	6			3			
UROLOGY	23	172	7.5			18	131	5	41	22		12	16
OPHTHALMOLOGY	5	18	3.6			3	9	2	9	5		2	2
RHINOLARYNG	5	17	3.4	1	1	3	13	1	3	5		1	1
ADULT T & A	2	4	2.0			2	4			2			
PED T & A	1	1	1.0	1	1					1			
PODIATRY	15	45	3.0			14	41	1	4	15		5	6
TOTALS INC / NB	650			83		484		83		547		277	
		4713	7.3		387		3366		960		8		428
LESS NEWBORNS	25	130											
TOTALS EXC / NB	625	4583											

TOTAL CASES	AVG. STAY	TRANSFERRED TO					LENGTH OF STAY DISTRIBUTION			
		OTHER HOSP.	SNF		HOME CARE		1 – 3 DAYS	4 – 14 DAYS	15 – 30 DAYS	OVER 30 DAYS
			UNDER 64	65 AND OVER	UNDER 64	65 AND OVER				
625	7.3	8	1	7			28%	62%	10%	%

% OF PATIENTS OPERATED	% OF EMERG ADM.	% OF PATIENTS W/ CONS	AVG. # OF CONS	TRANSFER RATE		
				TO OTHER HOSP.	TO SNF	TO HOME CARE
84%	01%	43%	2	1.2%	1.2%	

Figure 9.1.   **Computerized discharge analysis report** (*continued*)

HOSP # XXXX   JAN 20XX   PAGE 1

DISCHARGE STATUS							PAYMENT STATUS							
ALIVE STATUS	AMA	TRANSFER	DEATHS				COMMERCIAL		BLUE CROSS		MEDICAID		MEDICARE	
			EXP NO AUT	EXP AUT	COR. CASE									
					NO AUT	AUT	PAT.	DAYS	PAT.	DAYS	PAT.	DAYS	PAT.	DAYS
15	16	17	18	19	20	21	22	23	24	25	26	27	28	29
184	4	14	2				39	323	72	625	28	172	53	700
56		2	1	1			9	60	20	235	5	43	24	273
2											1	9	1	14
13							3	20	7	54	1	11	2	14
14			3				4	38	4	44	2	30	7	66
4							3	33			1	7		
		3					1	5	1	9			1	3
26							2	14	7	34	2	52		
9							1	1	1	1	6	20		
15							2	4	9	14	2	5		
33							7	22	16	51	10	52		
25							2	11	6	33	13	55		
47							12	73	16	91	18	100		
5							2	3	3	8				
5							3	19	1	7				
2									2	3				
1									1	2				
1											1	1		
33				1	1		11	57	19	107			4	38
6		1					2	22	2	21			3	31
76		1					29	233	20	161	8	21	4	46
4									3	7	1	1		
1							1	5						
3									3	6				
23							5	27	10	73	2	19	5	41
5									3	9			2	9
5							2	3	2	11			1	3
2									2	4				
1							1	1						
15							4	11	7	23	3	7	1	4
616		21		2				985		1633		605		1242
	4		7				145		237		114		108	

DEATHS						OTHER PAYMENT STATUS							
GROSS DEATH RATE	NET DEATH RATE	GROSS AUT. RATE	NET AUT. RATE	COR CASES	POST-OP	SELF-PAY		WORK-COMP		FREE OTHER – GOV		UMW	
						PAT	DAYS	PAT	DAYS	PAT	DAYS	PAT	DAYS
01%	01%	22%	22%			26	124	18	107	1	9		

DAY OF WEEK OF ADMISSION							DAY OF WEEK OF DISCHARGE						
SUN	MON	TUES	WED	THURS	FRI	SAT	SUN	MON	TUES	WED	THURS	FRI	SAT
13%	13%	18%	15%	17%	14%	10%	07%	12%	14%	19%	14%	19%	15%

Another verification can be done by adding the percentages given for the day-of-the-week admissions and the day-of-the-week discharges to make certain they add up to 100 percent. In the computerized statistical report in figure 9.1, they do add up to 100 percent (13 + 13 + 18 + 15 + 17 + 14 + 10 = 100, and 7 + 12 + 14 + 19 + 14 + 19 + 15 = 100). These data could be presented in the form of a **pie chart.** (See chapter 11.)

Reports such as the one shown in figure 9.1 are useful to hospital administrators; this type of review can give some insights into the resources and services used in the facility.

Example: The psychiatrists on staff are requesting that a new 15-bed psychiatry wing be built to accommodate their patients. The administrator could look at this report and see that there were only three psychiatry patients in this month. If this is normal for the hospital, then can the administration justify this expense? Most likely not. However, some other questions that could be posed by administration are: Would adding a separate psychiatry wing increase the number of admissions to the hospital? How many psychiatrists are in the community and would they admit their patients to our hospital if there were more beds? Is there something else happening in the community that could increase the number of psychiatry admissions? Are any of the psychiatry physician offices planning to add additional psychiatrists to the community?

Example: If the orthopedists asked for a new treatment room, the administrator can see that 77 patients were seen in this month and they have a fairly high length of stay. Certainly, additional comparison reports would need to be done to ascertain the number of patients seen by the orthopedists before a decision is made. Perhaps a more specific breakdown by age group and length of stay could help administration make a determination if more space is justified. However, these types of reports can serve as a baseline to begin collecting other types of data for decision-making projects.

Computerized Financial Statistical Reports

Computers are also used to compile various financial statistical reports. A sample computerized financial report is shown in figure 9.2.

Computerized Readmission Rate Reports

Figure 9.3 shows an example of a computerized readmission rate report. This type of report delineates inpatients by medical service and calculates each medical service's readmission rate.

Case-Mix Index Report

Figure 9.4 shows a sample of a computerized case-mix index report. This report portrays the facility's case-mix index for all financial classes for the month and the fiscal year to date. It also shows the case-mix index for Medicare-only patients. The **case-mix index** refers to the average relative weight of all cases treated at a given facility or by a given physician, which reflects the resource intensity or clinical severity of a specific group in relation to the other groups in the classification system. Case-mix is always reported with four decimal points. The formula for computing case-mix is:

$$\frac{\text{Sum of the weights of MS-DRGs (\textit{Medicare severity diagnosis-related groups})}}{\text{Total number of patients discharged}}$$

Figure 9.2.   Computerized financial report

	Community Hospital Most Frequent MS-DRGs by Financial Class Medicare Patients Only Annual Report, 20XX				
MS-DRG	**MS-DRG Title**	**No. of Pts**	**Pt. Days**	**ALOS**	**Tot. Charges**
293	Heart failure & shock w/o CC/MCC	216	1,252	5.8	$2,125,018.00
066	Intracranial hemorrhage or cerebral infarction w/o CC/MCC	141	1,009	7.2	$1,798,011.89
470	Major joint replacement or reattachment of lower extremity w/o MCC	136	926	6.8	$2,601,090.62
195	Simple pneumonia & pleurisy w/o CC/MCC	117	807	6.9	$1,271,445.45
192	Chronic obstructive pulmonary disease w/o CC/MCC	98	579	5.9	$920,071.41
378	G.I. hemorrhage w CC	94	487	5.2	$964,597.03
178	Respiratory infections & inflammations w CC	88	905	10.3	$1,656,856.52
330	Major small & large bowel procedures w CC	88	1,092	12.4	$2,493,260.52
391	Esophagitis, gastroent & misc digest disorders w MCC	86	324	3.8	$560,025.93
469	Major joint replacement or reattachment of lower extremity w MCC	81	617	7.6	$1,329,055.73
309	Cardiac arrhythmia & conduction disorders w CC	71	290	4.1	$506,803.44
311	Angina pectoris	70	234	3.3	$466,286.80
872	Septicemia w/o MV 96+ hours w/o MCC	69	619	9.0	$1,209,069.85
640	Nutritional & misc metabolic disorders w MCC	63	366	5.8	$532,230.77
286	Circulatory disorders except AMI, w card cath w MCC	56	248	4.4	$687,146.08
068	Nonspecific cva & precerebral occlusion w/o infarct w/o MCC	52	158	3.0	$336,667.38
280	Acute myocardial infarction, discharged alive w MCC	51	328	6.4	$790,417.76
689	Kidney & urinary tract infections w MCC	47	240	5.1	$367,789.93
189	Pulmonary edema & respiratory failure	43	369	8.6	$707,485.01
839	Chemo w acute leukemia as sdx w/o CC/MCC	41	85	2.1	$198,692.68
389	G.I. obstruction w CC	39	235	6.0	$386,509.40
244	Permanent cardiac pacemaker implant w/o CC/MCC	33	146	4.4	$592,506.88
394	Other digestive system diagnoses w CC	33	218	6.6	$427,499.12
315	Other circulatory system diagnoses w CC	31	189	6.1	$447,102.64

(continued on next page)

Figure 9.2.   Computerized financial report *(continued)*

	Community Hospital Most Frequent MS-DRGs by Financial Class Medicare Patients Only Annual Report, 20XX				
MS-DRG	**MS-DRG Title**	**No. of Pts**	**Pt. Days**	**ALOS**	**Tot. Charges**
208	Respiratory system diagnosis w ventilator support < 96 hours	31	387	12.5	$1,215,601.28
842	Lymphoma & non-acute leukemia w/o CC/MCC	1	4	4.0	$4,011.41
844	Other myeloprolif dis or poorly diff neopl diag w CC	1	23	23.0	$45,480.70
876	O.R. procedure w principal diagnoses of mental illness	1	20	20.0	$26,289.88
883	Disorders of personality & impulse control	1	19	19.0	$15,508.06
958	Other O.R. procedures for multiple significant trauma w CC	1	14	14.0	$35,775.10
913	Traumatic injury w MCC	1	4	4.0	$5,560.30
916	Allergic reactions w/o MCC	1	5	5.0	$10,687.30
922	Other injury, poisoning & toxic effect diag w MCC	1	2	2.0	$6,522.35
923	Other injury, poisoning & toxic effect diag w/o MCC	1	2	2.0	$3,161.58
941	O.R. proc w diagnoses of other contact w health services w/o CC/MCC	1	3	3.0	$3,302.98
947	Signs & symptoms w MCC	1	6	6.0	$9,279.07
264	Other circulatory system O.R. procedures	1	2	2.0	$23,031.87
956	Limb reattachment, hip & femur proc for multiple significant trauma	1	7	7.0	$21,149.70
959	Other O.R. procedures for multiple significant trauma w/o CC/MCC	1	5	5.0	$14,882.29
977	HIV w or w/o other related condition	1	4	4.0	$7,104.30
837	Other digestive system diagnoses w CC	1	10	10.0	$28,618.33
		1,891	**12,240**	**6.5**	**$24,851,607.34**

Figure 9.3.   Computerized readmission rate report

Community Hospital Readmission Rate For Month End 10/20XX			
Case Type	**Number of Readmits**	**Number of Cases**	**Readmit Rate (%)**
I	188	2,046	9.18

Readmission Rate by Service For Month End 10/20XX				
Case Type	**Medical Service**	**Number of Readmits**	**Number of Cases**	**Readmit Rate (%)**
I	ABS		3	0.00
I	ABT		1	0.00
I	ALL		1	0.00
I	CRD	10	277	3.61
I	CVS	10	84	11.90
I	DLC	5	70	7.14
I	DLN		16	0.00
I	DLR		53	0.00
I	END		2	0.00
I	FPR	5	75	6.66
I	GI	5	27	18.51
I	GYN	1	68	1.47
I	INF	1	8	12.50
I	MED	59	511	11.54
I	MON	26	67	38.80
I	NB	1	129	0.77
I	NEU	1	4	25.00
I	NIC		21	0.00
I	NIN		1	0.00
I	NPH	42	162	25.92
I	NRS		25	0.00
I	OB	3	80	3.75
I	ONR		1	0.00
I	OPH		1	0.00
I	ORS	2	14	14.28
I	ORT	4	84	4.76

(continued on next page)

Figure 9.3.   Computerized readmission rate report *(continued)*

Case Type	Medical Service	Number of Readmits	Number of Cases	Readmit Rate (%)
I	OTO		11	0.00
I	PED	1	55	1.81
I	PPA	1	2	50.00
I	PUL		4	0.00
I	RON	2	2	100.00
I	RPL		11	0.00
I	SUR	4	71	5.63
I	THS	3	37	8.10
I	URO	1	42	2.38
I	VSS	1	26	3.84
I			2,046	

Figure 9.4.   Computerized case-mix index report

Community Hospital Case-Mix Index Report—All Financial Classes For Fiscal Year to Date, 20XX		
Total Weight	**Number of Cases**	**Case-Mix Index**
6831.0912	3,230	2.1148
Case-Mix Index Report—Medicare Only For Fiscal Year to Date, 20XX		
Total Weight	**Number of Cases**	**Case-Mix Index**
2915.2882	1,367	2.1326
Case-Mix Index Report—All Financial Classes For Month End 10/20XX		
Total Weight	**Number of Cases**	**Case-Mix Index**
3396.8017	1,626	2.0890
Case-Mix Index Report—Medicare Only For Month End 10/20XX		
Total Weight	**Number of Cases**	**Case-Mix Index**
1364.1506	658	2.0731

Physician Reports

Healthcare organizations have always been interested in finding effective ways of measuring the utilization of services provided by physicians. One approach commonly used to analyze services is profiling. **Profiling** is defined as a measurement of the quality, utilization, and cost of medical resources provided by physicians that is made by employers, third-party payers, government entities, and other purchasers of healthcare. Figure 9.5 is a report of a facility's physician profile. This report lists important information about how physicians use the services of the facility. This is important to the organization's administration because they need to know if physician services are increasing or decreasing. If services are increasing, the question of additional equipment or staff needs to be addressed; if they are decreasing, the question of why becomes paramount.

Exercise 9.12

Complete the following exercises using the reports in figures 9.1 through 9.4.

1. The report in figure 9.1 gives the gross death rate (hospital death rate) as .01 percent. Recalculate this rate and round to the second decimal place.

2. Recalculate the gross autopsy rate in figure 9.1. Round your answer to the second decimal place.

3. In figure 9.2 which Medicare severity diagnosis-related group (MS-DRG) has the greatest ALOS?

4. Recalculate the readmission rates for the medical services and the overall rate in figure 9.3 to verify their accuracy. Which readmission rates were not accurate? Round your answers to two decimal points.

5. Recalculate the rates in figure 9.4 to verify their accuracy. Are there any that were calculated incorrectly? If so, which ones? How many Medicare patients were discharged during the fiscal year to date? At which month end was this report calculated?

Spreadsheets

Numerous statistical software packages are available for the creation of spreadsheets. **Spreadsheets,** or worksheets, allow you to enter text, numbers, and formulas to assist in calculations.

A spreadsheet consists of columns lettered across the top of the document and rows numbered down the left side of the document. The intersections of columns and rows form cells, which are the basic units for storing data.

Each software package varies slightly in method. Most packages perform basic arithmetic functions as well as many of the statistical calculations discussed in this book. Various add-in features allow for data sorting, formatting for printing data, and even graphical

Figure 9.5.   Physician profile

Atten. Phys.	Total							Deaths						Pts. Receiving Consults			
	Cases	Surg Cases	Days	ESD Pts.	ALOS	Preop LOS		TOT	% of Dths	Post Op	W/in 48 hrs	Aut Cas	Cor Cas	Tot Pts.	Cons Rec'd	Avg Cons	Cons Rate
01000	202	18	1,111	69	5.5	3.1		12	5.9	1		1		72	104	1.4	36%
01005	182	21	1,911	49	105.0	5.5		14	7.7		2	1		93	146	1.6	51%
01006	259	42	2,719	88	10.3	4.5		15	5.8	2	2	1		122	175	1.4	47%
01009	242	29	2,250	79	9.3	3.8		18	7.4	1	3	1	1	117	162	1.4	48%
04000	53	6	509	9	9.6	4.0		4	7.5		1			30	43	1.4	57%
10125	1	1	2		2.0	1.0											
15000	3	3	31	1	10.3	1.0								1	1	1.0	33%
15002	76	10	737	19	9.7	4.6		4	5.3		1	1		55	93	1.7	72%
15006	188	18	1,354	64	7.2	5.6		7	3.7	1	1	1	1	77	103	1.3	41%
15007	2		18	2	9.0												
15008	95	5	751	32	7.9	4.0		4	4.2			2		55	76	1.4	58%
Total	**1,303**	**153**	**11,393**	**412**	**8.7**	**3.7**		**78**	**6.0**	**5**	**10**	**8**	**2**	**622**	**903**	**1.4**	**48%**

interface. Most software packages contain a help section and a tutorial to assist the novice. The best way to gain proficiency with any software package is to "just do it" and practice, practice, practice.

Exercise 9.13

Complete the following spreadsheets.

1. Using Worksheet No. 1 in exercise 3.9 on page 36, create a computerized spreadsheet to calculate the patient census.

2. Using the table in exercise 5.4 on page 62, which lists 15 patients by name, age, clinical service, and LOS, create a computerized spreadsheet to calculate the ALOS.

Chapter 9 Test

Complete the following exercises.

1. If your HIM department has 100,000 active medical records and you received 5,352 requests for records within a six-month period, what is the request rate for the past six months? Round to two decimal points.

2. Of the 5,352 requests for medical records in the question above, 4,257 were located within the 20-minute time frame established by the supervisor as a quality improvement indicator. What is the rate of compliance in answering requests for records? Round to two decimal points.

3. Community Health Center, a new patient clinic in your town serving only underinsured and uninsured patients, has asked you to help its HIM department get started. Calculate the number of new shelving units needed for a medical record filing system based on eight shelves per unit at 36 inches per shelf. The average record size equals 0.30 inches, and the center anticipates seeing 4,500 patients the first year.

4. After one month of operation, the health information services at Community Health Center determined that there were two records misfiled out of the 450 active records. What is the filing accuracy rate for this area? Round to one decimal point.

5. An employee currently earning $13.85 per hour has been awarded a 3.5 percent merit raise. What will the employee's hourly salary be with this increase?

6. It takes approximately 15 minutes to code one record. How many personnel hours would be needed to code 1,424 discharges for the month?

(continued on next page)

Chapter 9 Test (continued)

7. A coding supervisor must determine the number of full-time equivalents (FTEs) needed to code 500 discharges per week. If it takes an average of 20 minutes to code each record and each coder works 7.5 productive hours per day, how many FTEs will the coding supervisor need? (Round to one decimal place.)

8. The HIM department at Community Hospital will experience a 15 percent increase in the number of discharges coded per day as the result of opening a cardiac clinic in the facility. The 15 percent increase is projected to be 100 additional records per day. The standard time to code this type of record is 10 minutes. Compute the number of FTEs required to handle this increased volume in coding based on a seven-hour productive day. Round to one digit after the decimal.

9. The HIM coding supervisor agrees to pay a new graduate $13.50 per hour. This is a full-time coding position at 2,080 hours per year. The cost for a full-time employee's fringe benefits is 24 percent of the employee's salary. How much must the supervisor budget for the employee's salary and fringe benefits?

10. The same supervisor in the scenario above agreed to increase the salary of the employee to $15.00 per hour once she passed her RHIT exam. Three months after beginning her employment, the employee passed her RHIT exam. What will the new budget be for salary and fringe benefits?

11. The forms used in your coding area cost $100.00 per 1,000 forms for the first 2,000 and $50 for every 1,000 thereafter. If you need to order 5,000 forms, what is the total cost?

12. You currently lease scanning equipment at a cost of $1,500 per quarter and two copy machines at $120 each per month. What will you need to budget annually for this leased equipment?

13. What is the variance and percent of variance for each item listed in the HIM department budget shown in the table below? Round to two decimal points.

Community Hospital
Health Information Department
Fiscal Year 20XX

Item	Budget Amount	Actual Amount	Variance/% of Variance
Supplies	$1,600	$1,595	
Outside temp service	$6,800	$7,200	
Travel	$1,500	$1,526	
Conference fees	$500	$455	
Postage	$1,000	$1,017	
Subscriptions	$325	$330	
Maintenance contracts	$1,500	$1,500	

Chapter 9 Test (continued)

14. All the patients who present to the emergency services department with a suspected acute myocardial infarction (AMI) are expected to receive an ECG within 10 minutes of their arrival. Of the 56 patients who had a suspected AMI during the last quarter, 32 had an ECG within the specified time frame. What was the rate of compliance? Round to two decimal places.

15. Last month, the release of information specialist received 232 requests for information. He was able to answer 176 within the specified time frame of three working days. What is the rate of compliance in answering requests within the specified time frame? Round to two decimal places.

16. Estimate the hospital charges for the patients listed in the table below based on an average cost of $950 per day.

Community Hospital

Patient Number	LOS	Estimated Charges
171819	3	
124785	4	
452362	5	
326578	8	
528615	9	
213624	12	
242628	10	
659832	5	
428231	3	
269761	5	

17. Last year, Community Hospital had 23,652 admissions. Of these, 1,569 were readmissions. What is the hospital's readmission rate? Round to two decimal places.

18. In September, the hospital had three coders who coded 1,200 inpatient records, and 18 of the records failed the quality screens.
    a. What is the average number of records coded by each coder?
    b. What was the average number of records coded each working day (Monday through Friday at 21 workdays) in September? Round to two decimal points.
    c. What percentage of records passed the quality screens? Round to two decimal points.

(continued on next page)

Chapter 9 Test (continued)

19. At Community Hospital each full-time employee is required to work 2,080 hours annually. The table below shows the amount of time that five employees were absent from work over the past year. Use this information to answer the following questions. Round all answers to two decimal places.

    a. What is the total absentee rate for each employee?
    b. What is the sick leave rate for each employee?
    c. What is the total sick leave rate for this group of employees for the year?

Community Hospital
Health Information Management Department
Coding Section
Absentee Report
Annual Statistics, 20XX

Employee Name	Vacation Hours Used	Sick Leave Hours Used
A	40	0
B	20	16
C	32	8
D	80	32
E	16	40

20. The coding department of a large physician clinic is interested in purchasing a software program that will edit claims before they are sent to the Billing Office. The license fee for the software is $52,000 per year. The software is expected to reduce the number of errors on claims and thus reduce the number of claims returned to the clinic for recoding. Currently, the department codes 32,600 physician visits per month and 450 claims are returned each month for recoding. The facility pays two FTEs in the Billing Office $11.50 per hour each (plus 25 percent benefits) to refile the returned claims. The software company promises that its software will reduce the number of returned claims by 90 percent.

    a. What is the rate of claims that are currently being returned for recoding each month? Round to two decimal places.
    b. How many claims would be returned after the installation of the software?
    c. If the clinic eliminated the two FTEs that handle the returned claims, what savings would it realize after installation of the software?
    d. What is the payback period?
    e. What is the return on investment?

Chapter 9 Test (continued)

21. What is physician profiling, and why is it important to healthcare organizations?

22. Spreadsheet software programs allow you to enter text, numbers, and formulas to assist in calculations. True or false?

23. What is a hospital's case-mix index?

24. Using the information in the table below, calculate the case-mix index for each month in the first quarter at Community Hospital. (Round to four decimal places.)

Community Hospital
First Quarter Statistics, 20XX
Case-Mix Report

	January	February	March
Total discharges	2,012	1,983	2,112
Total weight	7156.2315	7733.7523	9715.2354
Case-mix index			

Chapter 10
Descriptive Statistics in Healthcare

Key Terms

Decile	Normal distribution of data
Descriptive statistics	Outlier
Frequency distribution	Quartile
Graph	Range
Measurements	Skewness
Measures of central tendency	Standard deviation
Mean	Variability
Median	Variable
Mode	Variance

Objectives

At the conclusion of this chapter, you should be able to:

- Define descriptive statistics
- Define the terms rank, quartile, decile, and percentile
- Explain how and why percentiles are used
- Compute the percentile from an ungrouped distribution
- Define and compute the mean, median, and mode
- Define and differentiate among range, variance, and standard deviation
- Calculate range, variance, and standard deviation
- Define and compute correlation

Descriptive Statistics

Descriptive statistics are used to describe data in ways that are manageable and easily understood. The following sections discuss the basic concepts of rank, quartile, decile, percentile, measures of central tendency (mean, median, mode), measures of variation (range, variance, standard deviation), and correlation.

Frequency Distribution

Before studying measures in descriptive statistics, it would be useful to briefly cover two concepts: **variable** and **frequency distribution.** A variable is a characteristic that can have different values. For example, a person may be HIV negative or positive. The characteristic or variable is HIV status and the values are negative and positive. Third-party payers, race, LOS, and services are examples of variables. Within each variable, there is more than one possible value. For example, third-party payers include numerous insurance companies. The variable is "third-party payer" while the values are the names of the organizations paying for services.

Because it is difficult to draw conclusions from data in raw form, they are often summarized into frequency distributions. A frequency distribution shows the values that a variable can take and the number of observations associated with each value. Using the previous example, a facility conducting HIV testing may be interested in the number or frequency of HIV negative and positive individuals using their services. This information is valuable when seeking funding.

Example: Table 10.1 provides an example of a frequency distribution in which types of third-party payers are identified, along with the number of patients in an organization associated with each payer.

Rank

Rank denotes a value's position in a group relative to other values organized in order of magnitude. For example, a rank of 50 means that a value or score is 50th from the beginning (or end) of a series. The number of scores in a sequence is important in determining

Table 10.1.   Example of a frequency distribution by number of patients discharged from community hospital by third-party payer, June 20XX

Third-Party Payer	No. of Patients
Medicare	98
Medicaid	56
Tri-Care	23
Blue Cross	85
Mutual of Omaha	67
Other Private Payer	76
Total	**405**

the significance of a rank. If there are only 60 scores, a rank of 50th is interpreted much differently than if there are 1,000 scores. For this reason, it may be more useful to express data as percentiles.

In ranked data, the position of the observation is more important than the number associated with it. For example, it is possible to list the major causes of death in the United States, along with the number of lives that each cause claimed. If the causes were ordered starting with the one that resulted in the greatest number of deaths and ending with the one that caused the fewest, and these were assigned consecutive integers, the data are said to be ranked.

Table 10.2 shows a report listing the 15 leading causes of death in the United States for the latest data available (2007). Note that cerebrovascular disease would be ranked third regardless of whether it caused 562,874 or 135,953 deaths.

Quartile

In addition to determining the rank of the score in a group, it can be helpful to divide data into parts to better understand the relationship among scores. Data organized in order of magnitude can be divided into four equal parts, or **quartiles.** The first quartile corresponds to the 25th percentile and includes the first 25 percent of the data, the second quartile corresponds to the 50th percentile and includes 50 percent of the data, and so on.

Table 10.2.   **Fifteen leading causes of death in the United States in 2007**

Rank	Causes of Death	Total Deaths
1	Diseases of heart	616,067
2	Malignant neoplasms	562,875
3	Cerebrovascular diseases	135,952
4	Chronic lower respiratory diseases	127,924
5	Accidents (unintentional injuries)	123,706
6	Alzheimer's disease	74,632
7	Diabetes mellitus	71,382
8	Influenza and pneumonia	52,717
9	Nephritis, nephritic syndrome, and nephrosis	46,448
10	Septicemia	34,828
11	Intentional self-harm (suicide)	34,598
12	Chronic liver disease and cirrhosis	29,165
13	Essential hypertension and hypertensive renal disease	23,965
14	Parkinson's disease	20,058
15	Assault (homicide)	18,361

Source: CDC, FastStats, http://www.cdc.gov/nchs/fastats/lcod.htm.

Decile

In similar fashion, **deciles** represent data divided into 10 equal parts. The first decile corresponds to the 10th percentile and includes the first 10% of the scores, the second decile corresponds to the 20th percentile and includes the second 10% of the data, and so on.

Percentile

As quartiles divide scores into four equal parts and deciles into 10, percentiles separate the scores into 100 equal parts. If a person scores at the 54th percentile, his score is greater than or equal to 54% of all the scores in the group. This is called a percentile rank.

How and Why Percentiles Are Used

Percentiles help people understand their score relative to all scores from a group. If a student is told that she received a score of 34 on a test and she did not know how many points were possible, the 34 has no significance. However, if she is told that the score was in the 95th percentile, this would give a better understanding of the score compared to her peers; that is, only 5% of the class received a higher score.

To find the score that falls within a given percentile in a group of data arranged in order of magnitude:

1. Multiply the desired percentile's percentage by the total number of scores in the given group of scores (N). For example, the 38th percentile's percentage would be 38%. Likewise, the 90th percentile's percentage would be 90%.

2. This number indicates the rank of the score in the group that represents the desired percentile.

Example: The following numbers represent lengths of newborns in inches.

12, 12, 12, 13, 13, 15, 15, 16, 17, 18, 19, 20, 21, 21, 22, 22, 23, 23, 24, 25

$$N = 20$$

To find the 60th percentile:

1. Multiply 60% by 20 (N) = 12

2. Count up to the 12th score

3. The 60th percentile is 20

This means that 40% of the newborns were over 20 inches in length at birth.

On the other hand, if you want to know in what percentile a score is, take that score and divide the number of scores that are equal to and less than your score by the total number of scores and then multiply by 100.

Example: For instance, in the example above, suppose you want to find the percentile of the newborns that are over 17 inches in length. Take 9 (17 is the ninth score) divided by 20 (the N) × 100.

$$\left(\frac{9}{20}\right) \times 100 = 45^{th} \text{ percentile}$$

17 falls in the 45th percentile. This means that 45% of the newborns were 17 inches or less in length at birth and 55% (100% − 45%) were over 17 inches in length at birth.

Exercise 10.1

1. Your instructor told you that you are in the 54th percentile in your class. This means that your score is greater than or equal to 54% of all the scores in the class. True or false?

2. Use the information below to find your percentile. Your score is 86.

Test Scores out of 100 Points

95	97
99	74
84	91
65	94
54	89
35	88
86	56
77	96
76	27
100	75
92	93

Measures of Central Tendency

In summarizing data, it is often useful to have a single number that is representative of the entire collection of data or specific population. Such numbers are customarily referred to as **measures of central tendency.** A common measure of central tendency is average or mean. It is the sum of a set of numbers divided by the number of data points. One of the most common examples of a mean or average in a healthcare facility involves average length of stay, or ALOS (average number of days from admission to discharge that patients stay in the hospital). The ALOS was discussed in detail in chapter 5 and is discussed briefly in this chapter.

Three measures of central tendency are frequently used: mean, median, and mode. Each measure has advantages and disadvantages in describing a typical value.

Mean

The **mean** is the arithmetic average. It is common to use the term average to designate mean. It is computed by dividing the sum of all the scores (Σ) by the total number of scores (N).

Example: Seven hospital inpatients have the following lengths of stay: 2, 3, 4, 3, 5, 1, and 3 days. To construct a frequency distribution, all the values that the LOS can take are listed in ascending order (in this example, 1, 2, 3, 4, and 5) and the number of times a discharged patient had each LOS is entered. Table 10.3 shows the frequency distribution for this example. As the table shows, three patients were discharged with an LOS of three days each and the remaining four patients were discharged with an LOS of one, two, four, and five days each.

Table 10.3.   **Frequency distribution of seven hospital inpatients**

LOS	No. of Patients Discharged
1	1
2	1
3	3
4	1
5	1

To obtain the mean, divide the total number of inpatient days $(1 + 2 + 3 + 3 + 3 + 4 + 5 = 21)$ by the number of values (or frequency distribution), in this case, seven inpatients. This gives a mean of three days. This may also be written as mean $(\overline{X}) = 3$ days.

The symbol $\overline{X}$ (pronounced "ex bar") is used to represent the mean in this formula

$$\frac{Total\ sum\ of\ all\ the\ values}{Number\ of\ values\ involved} = \overline{X}$$

or

$$\frac{\Sigma\ scores}{N} = \frac{Sum\ of\ all\ scores}{Total\ number\ of\ scores}$$

Handy Tip: You may hear individuals refer to the average or mean as "The average age is 10 to 20." This is the wrong use of this statistic. In this example, they are referring to a range of ages, which may be the desired expression in some instances. However, the average is only one value.

The mean is the most common measure of central tendency. One of its advantages is that it is easy to compute. It is used as the basis for a large proportion of statistical tests. One disadvantage of the mean is that it is sensitive to extreme values called **outliers** that may distort its representation of the central tendency of a set of numbers. For example, if six women in a group weighed 110, 115, 120, 122, 125, and 227 pounds, the mean weight of the group would be $\frac{819}{6}$, or 136.5 pounds. However, given that five of the women weigh 125 pounds or less, the mean of this sample is not a very good indication of central tendency. Thus, the more asymmetric or unequal the distribution, the less desirable it is to summarize the observations by using the mean.

Median

The **median** is the midpoint (center) of the distribution of values, or the point above and below which 50 percent of the values fall. The median value is obtained by arranging the numerical observations in ascending or descending order and then determining the middle value. This may be the middle observation (if there is an odd number of values) or a point halfway between the two middle values (if there is an even number of values).

To arrive at the median in an even-numbered distribution, add the two middle values together and divide by 2. When the two middle values are the same, the median is that value.

Example: The numbers in the LOS example used earlier are sequenced as follows:

1

2

3

3 ← median (midpoint)

3

4

5

The median is 3.

Example: The median weight of the women who weighed 110, 115, 120, 122, 125, and 227 pounds is shown as follows:

110

115

120

$\leftarrow$ median $\left(120 + 122 = \dfrac{242}{2} = 121\right)$

122

125

227

The median is 121.

Handy Tip: The advantage to using the median as a measure of central tendency is that it is unaffected by outliers. The value of 121 pounds is much more representative of the fact that five out of the six women weigh 125 pounds or less than the mean value of 136.5 as seen in the previous example.

The median is also often used in calculating length of stay in long-term care cases. As discussed in chapter 5, a long-stay patient's discharge days are allocated to the period in which he or she is discharged. Sometimes this can give a distorted average, especially on a monthly (rather than annual) basis.

Example: In March, a long-term care facility discharged 130 patients with a total length of stay of 1,267 days. The LOS for one of the patients was 365 days. The ALOS for all 130 patients was 9.8 days ($\frac{1,267}{130}$ = 9.75). If the stay of the one patient is removed from the total length of stay, the ALOS becomes 6.99 or 7.0 days (1,267 − 365 = $\frac{902}{129}$ = 6.99). Should one patient or a few patients in a population affect the average to this degree? Is the statistical computation meaningful for decision-making purposes? In this situation, the facility has two options:

- First, a notation can be made on the report that either the ALOS of 9.8 includes one patient who stayed 365 days or the ALOS of 7.0 excludes one patient who stayed 365 days. Both calculations can be made. Appropriate notes should be attached to the report to indicate the difference.

- Second, the computation using the median rather than the mean can be used. The individual lengths of stay would be arranged in numerical order from highest to lowest, or vice versa.

Median Used to Describe Length of Stay

The list in Table 10.4 includes the LOS of 15 discharged patients.

These numbers placed in order from highest to lowest are: 28, 21, 9, 8, 5, 5, 4, 4, 4, 4, 3, 2, 2, 2, and 1. The midpoint falls at 4. Note that, regardless of value, 50 percent of the total numbers fall above this point and 50 percent fall below. The median provides a more revealing representation of the ALOS when one or a few long-stay patients would otherwise distort the arithmetic mean. The median is not sensitive to outliers as is the mean. However, one disadvantage of using the median is that manual computation is much more time-consuming than computation of the mean. Moreover, it would be impractical with a large number of discharged patients. If the statistical computation is manual, it would be better to use the mean. However, if the statistical computation is computerized, it would be better to use the median.

According to Table 10.4, patients on the clinical medicine service stayed 28, 8, 5, 5, 4, 4 and 2 days for a total of 56 days. Using the formula, the ALOS for medicine patients is 8.0 days. The median, or midpoint, is 5. One patient had a long stay of 28 days. If that patient is removed from the calculation, the ALOS for medicine patients would be 4.7 days. In this case, the median would be a better choice to show the ALOS for these patients.

Mode

Mode is the third measure of central tendency and is the value that occurs most frequently in the data. In this sense, it is the value that is most typical. Its advantage is that it is the simplest of the measures of central tendency because it does not require any calculations. Referring to the first example above, the mode would be 3 because 3 is the most frequent value in the set.

Table 10.4.   LOS of 15 discharged patients

Name	Age	Clinical Service	Admission Date	Length of Stay
Adams	23	Medicine	6/01	4
Baldridge	68	Medicine	5/28	8
Carpenter	62	Medicine	6/01	4
Davis	12	Medicine	5/08	28
Edison	56	Surgery	6/01	4
Faison	87	Medicine	5/31	5
Garsten	19	Obstetrics	6/03	2
Halstead	35	Obstetrics	6/01	4
Isben	67	Medicine	6/03	2
Jackson	54	Surgery	5/15	21
Kaspan	29	Obstetrics	6/03	2
Lorenzo	78	Medicine	5/31	5
Martin	42	Obstetrics	6/02	3
Nasbin	32	Obstetrics	6/04	1
Ottoperin	98	Surgery	5/27	9
Total				**102**

While the mode is simple to use, there are disadvantages to using it. In the case of a small number of values, each value could occur only once and there will be no mode. Or, two values may be more common than others and you could have two or more modes.

Handy Tip: The mode does not have to be numerical. If you ask every person in your class what his or her favorite food is and tally the answers, you will most likely find a mode.

Example: Add another patient's LOS of 35 to the LOS example on page 177 to illustrate the mean and the median. The values would now total 56 (1 + 2 + 3 + 3 + 4 + 5 + 35). Divide 56 by the number of values involved (8) to calculate the mean of 7, or $\frac{56}{8} = 7$.

The median would be calculated as follows:

1

2

3

3

$\leftarrow$ median $\left(3 + 3 = \frac{6}{2} = 3\right)$

3

4

5

35

The median is 3, and the mode remains at 3.

This example shows that the median and the mode can be unaffected by extreme values.

The mode is rarely used as a sole descriptive measure of central tendency because it may not be unique; there may be two or more modes. These are called bimodal (two modes) or multimodal (several modes) distributions.

Example: The following represents a collection of values of lengths of stay:

1

1

1

2

2

3

3

3

4

5

5

5

7

9

In this group of patients, the modes for the LOS are 1, 3, and 5. The mode is the score that occurs most frequently; in this example, it occurred three times in 1, 3, and 5.

The choice of a measure of central tendency depends on the number of values and the nature of their distribution. Occasionally the mean, median, and mode are identical. For statistical analyses, however, the mean is preferable, whenever possible, because it includes information from all observations. However, if the series of values contains a few that are unusually high or low, the median may represent the series better than the mean. The mode is often used in samples where the most typical value is preferred.

Exercise 10.2

Complete the following exercises.

1. Fourteen patients have the following LOS: 1, 4, 4, 2, 5, 16, 3, 3, 1, 6, 4, 5, 7, and 2. Compute the mean, median, and mode.

2. A student's 10 scores on 10-point class quizzes include a 6, a 7, a 4, five 9s, an 8, and a 10. The student claims that her average grade on quizzes is 9 because most of her scores are 9s. Is this correct? Explain.

3. Last month, 10 patients between the ages of 11 and 13 were seen in their pediatrician's clinic. Their heights were recorded as 50, 56, 59, 51, 53, 51, 50, 52, 54 and 51 inches. Determine the mean, median, and mode.

4. Fourteen patients have the following LOS: 2, 3, 4, 1, 4, 16, 4, 2, 1, 5, 4, 3, 6, and 1. Calculate the mean, median, and mode.

5. An HIM supervisor timed his staff for eight hours during the workday to determine the average number of inpatient records coded in one hour. Using the findings listed below, what were the mean, median, and mode for each coder? What were the overall mean, median, and mode for the coding section? Round the mean to one decimal place.

Community Hospital
HIM Department
Number of Records Coded

Coder A		Coder B		Coder C		Coder D	
Hour 1	4	Hour 1	4	Hour 1	6	Hour 1	5
Hour 2	3	Hour 2	4	Hour 2	5	Hour 2	5
Hour 3	5	Hour 3	5	Hour 3	2	Hour 3	4
Hour 4	2	Hour 4	2	Hour 4	3	Hour 4	4
Hour 5	6	Hour 5	3	Hour 5	5	Hour 5	3
Hour 6	5	Hour 6	5	Hour 6	5	Hour 6	3
Hour 7	3	Hour 7	5	Hour 7	3	Hour 7	4
Hour 8	3	Hour 8	3	Hour 8	2	Hour 8	2

Answers:

Coder A:

Coder B:

Coder C:

Coder D:

Overall:

Measures of Variation

Measures of central tendency are not the only statistics used to summarize a frequency distribution. A facility also may want to consider the spread of the distribution, or the measure of variation. The measure of variation shows how widely the observations are spread out around the measure of central tendency. The mean gives a measure of central tendency of a list of numbers but tells nothing about the spread of the numbers in the list.

Example: Review the following three groups:

Group A	3	5	6	3	3
Group B	4	4	4	4	4
Group C	10	1	0	0	9

Each of these groups has a mean of 4 ($\frac{20}{5}$), and yet it is clear that the amount of dispersion or variation within the groups is different. The measures of spread increase with greater variation in the values in the frequency distribution. The spread is equal to zero when there is no variation, for example, when all the values in a frequency distribution are the same, as shown in group B.

Variability

Variability refers to the difference between each score and every other score. For example, if there are 100 scores, you would have to compute the difference between the first score and each of the 99 other scores, and then compute the difference between the second score and each of the 98 remaining scores, and so on. There would be 4,950 differences in all. A more feasible approach, which serves the purpose equally well, is to define the differences or deviations for all the scores in terms of how far each is from the average or the mean.

Range

The **range** is the simplest measure of spread. It indicates the difference between the largest and smallest values in a frequency distribution. In reviewing the three groups in the previous section on variability, the largest number in group A is 6 and the smallest is 3, a difference of 3. In group B, the difference is 0, and in group C, the difference is 10. Therefore, the range for group A is 3, the range for group B is 0, and the range for group C is 10.

Range has the advantage of being easy to compute. It is the simplest order-based measure of spread, but it is far from optimal as a measure of variability for two reasons. First, as the sample size increases, the range also tends to increase. Second, it is obviously affected by extreme values that are very different from other values in the data.

Exercise 10.3

Complete the following exercises.

1. Fourteen patients have the following LOS: 2, 3, 3, 1, 4, 18, 3, 2, 1, 5, 4, 3, 6, and 1. What is the range of this distribution of numbers?

2. Find the range in the following sets:

    a. 4, 3, 7, 15, 6, 8
    b. 0, –1, 8, 15, –4, 7.65
    c. 85, 91, 127, 76, 42, 47

3. The range in a frequency distribution is 22. If the lowest value is 3, what is the highest value?

4. The range in a frequency distribution is 54. If the highest value is 107, what is the lowest value?

5. A group of women seen at a diabetes clinic weighed 145, 127, 209, 216, 154, 165, 174, and 227 pounds. What is the range?

Because the range is determined by the two extremes only, a preferable measure of variability would include the distribution of all the values, not just those at the extremes. More informative measures of variation are variance and standard deviation.

Variance

The **variance** of a frequency distribution is the average of the standard deviations from the mean. The symbol s^2 is used to show the variance of a sample. "The variance of a distribution is larger when the observations are widely spread" (Johns 2011, 532). The formula for calculating the variance is:

$$s^2 = \frac{(X_1 - \overline{X})^2 + (X_2 - \overline{X})^2 + (X_3 - \overline{X})^2 \text{ and so on}}{N - 1}$$

Or you could use the notation of

$$s^2 = \frac{\Sigma(X - \overline{X})^2}{N - 1}$$

To calculate the variance, first determine the mean. Then, the squared deviations from the mean are calculated by subtracting the mean from each value in the distribution. The difference between the two values is squared $(X - \overline{X})^2$. The squared differences are summed and divided by $N - 1$.

s^2 = variance

Σ = sum

X = value of a measure or observation

$\overline{X}$ = mean

N = number of values or observations

$N - 1$ is used in the denominator instead of N to adjust for the fact that the mean of the sample is used as an estimate of the mean of the underlying population.

The more the values in a distribution are different from one another, the greater the variance and standard deviation. On page 181, the variance in group B equals 0 because all the values are the same. Measures of variation equal zero when there is no variation.

Example: Calculate the variance using the previous data: a sample of fourteen patients has the following LOS: 2, 3, 3, 1, 4, 18, 3, 2, 1, 5, 4, 3, 6, and 1. In the next computation, $\overline{X}$ is the actual LOS per patient. The mean LOS is calculated as follows:

$$\frac{56}{14} = 4 \text{ days}$$

The order of this computation is as follows:

1. Subtract the mean from each LOS score (enter result in column 3).

2. Square each result (enter result in column 4).

3. Add columns 3 and 4.

4. Divide column 4 by $(N - 1)$.

The variance is computed as follows:

$$s^2 = \frac{(2-4)^2 + (3-4)^2 + (3-4)^2 + (1-4)^2 + (4-4)^2 \text{ and so on}}{(14-1)} = \frac{240}{13} = 18.46$$

Column 1	Column 2	Column 3	Column 4
		LOS – Mean (4)	(LOS – Mean)²
Patient	**Length of Stay**	$(X - \overline{X})$	$(X - \overline{X})^2$
1	2	–2	4
2	3	–1	1
3	3	–1	1
4	1	–3	9
5	4	0	0
6	18	14	196
7	3	–1	1
8	2	–2	4
9	1	–3	9
10	5	1	1
11	4	0	0
12	3	–1	1
13	6	2	4
14	1	–3	9
Total	**56**	**0**	**240**

In this example, the size of the variance is influenced by the one LOS of 18 days. The more the values in a distribution are different from each other, the greater the variance and standard deviation.

Handy Tip: The sum of the deviations from the mean is always equal to zero. Therefore, by squaring the differences from the mean, the negative and positive deviations do not cancel each other out. When they are squared, negative as well as positive values become positive.

Standard Deviation

The **standard deviation (SD)** is the square root of the variance. As such, it can be more easily interpreted as a measure of variation. If the SD is small, there is less dispersion around the mean. If the SD is large, there is greater dispersion around the mean.

Handy Tip: The square root of a number is that number whose square is the number. The square of a number is that number multiplied by itself. For example, the square root of 9 is 3 ($3 \times 3 = 9$).

To understand this concept, it is helpful to learn about what mathematicians call normal distribution of data. A **normal distribution of data** means that most of the values in a set of data are close to the "average" and relatively few values tend to one extreme or the other, creating a bell-shaped distribution curve.

The SD is a statistic that tells how closely all the observations are clustered around the mean in a set of data. When the examples are closely gathered and the bell-shaped curve is steep, the SD is small. When the examples are spread apart and the bell-shaped curve is relatively flat, the SD is relatively large.

Therefore, normal distribution means that if the variable of a particular characteristic for every member of the population were measured, the frequency distribution would display a normal pattern, with most of the **measurements** near the center of the frequency. It also would be possible to accurately describe the population, with respect to a variable, by calculating the mean, variance, and SD of the values.

> **Example:** Computing the value of a standard deviation can be complicated. Figure 10.1 shows an example of a normal distribution. The center, or mean, is at 6. The SD in this example is 2.45. This means that about 68 percent of the observations in the frequency distribution fall within 2.45 standard deviations of 6 (6 ± 2.45). Thus, 68 percent fall between 3.55 and 8.45; approximately 95 percent fall between 1.1 and 10.9; and 99.7 percent fall between −1.35 and 13.35.

The formula for calculating standard deviation is:

$$SD = \sqrt{\frac{\sum (X - \overline{X})^2}{(N-1)}}$$

Figure 10.1.   Example of normal distribution

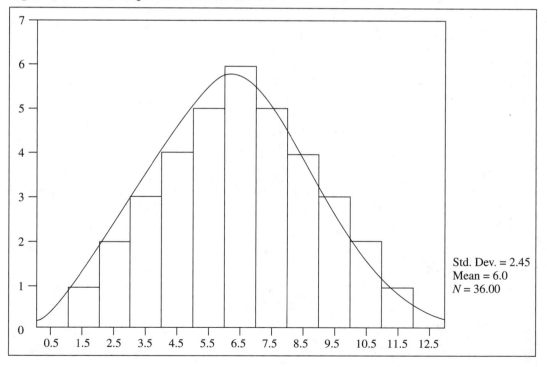

Std. Dev. = 2.45
Mean = 6.0
N = 36.00

Example: Continuing with the LOS example on page 183, the mean is 4 and the variance is 18.46. Thus, the SD is 4.3 (the square root of 18.46 = 4.30).

This means that ±1 SD contains values ranging from –0.3 to 8.3 (to get these figures add 1 SD to the mean of 4 so ±1 SD = 4 – 4.3 to 4 + 4.3 = –0.3 to 8.3).

±2 SD includes values ranging from –4.6 to 12.6 (to get these figures add 2 SD to the mean of 4 so ±2 SD = 4 – 8.6 to 4 + 8.6 = –4.6 to 12.6).

And ±3 SD includes all values ranging from –8.9 to 16.9.

Figure 10.2 shows a **graph** of standard deviation of the LOS example.

Example: In evaluating the LOS data, one can conclude that 13 out of 14 (92.9%) LOS fell within ±1 SD from the mean. The remaining value, 18, falls outside the ±3 SD from the mean and is called an outlier.

It should be noted that the distribution above is not a normal distribution. As stated earlier, in a normal distribution, one SD in both directions from the mean contains 68.3 percent of all values. In this data set, approximately 93 percent of the scores fall between ±1 SD from the mean. Visual inspection of the data in the LOS example reveals a fairly homogeneous data set despite the large SD. This emphasizes the importance of visual inspection of the data set when making decisions based on statistical calculations.

Figure 10.2.   Example of standard deviation

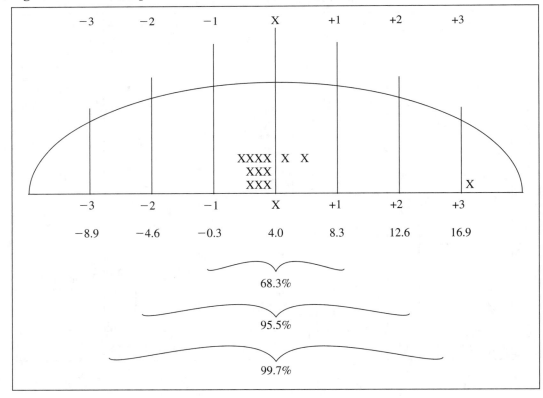

Source: Huffman.

Exercise 10.4

The following sample report from a cancer registry shows the SDs of weights for 20 males with adenocarcinoma of the rectum. Validate the calculations used in the report.

Weights of Males with Adenocarcinoma of Rectum

Patient	Weight lbs. (X)	$(X - \overline{X})$	$(X - \overline{X})^2$
1	142	−30	900
2	148	−24	576
3	151	−21	441
4	155	−17	289
5	155	−17	289
6	158	−14	196
7	164	−8	64
8	165	−7	49
9	170	−2	4
10	173	1	1
11	175	3	9
12	175	3	9
13	175	3	9
14	183	11	121
15	185	13	169
16	186	14	196
17	189	17	289
18	193	21	441
19	198	26	676
20	200	28	784
Total	**20**	**3,440**	**0**	**5,512**

*$SD = 17.0$; $s^2 = \frac{5,512}{19} = 290.1$; mean = 172; and $N - 1 = 19$

Not all distributions are symmetrical or have the usual bell-shaped curve. Some curves are skewed; that is, their numbers do not fall in the middle but, rather, on one end of the curve. **Skewness** is the horizontal stretching of a frequency distribution to one side or the other so that one tail is longer than the other. The direction of skewness is on the side of the long tail. Thus, if the longer tail is on the right, the curve is skewed to the right. If the longer tail is on the left, the curve is skewed to the left. (See figures 10.3 and 10.4.)

Figure 10.3.   Example of a curve skewed to the right (positive skew)

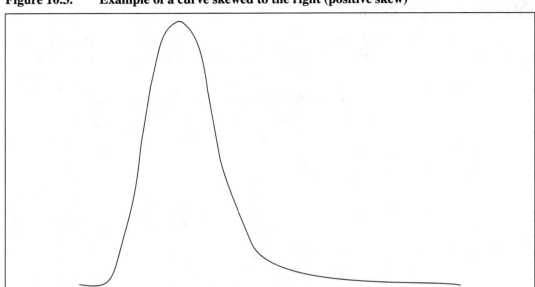

Figure 10.4.   Example of a curve skewed to the left (negative skew)

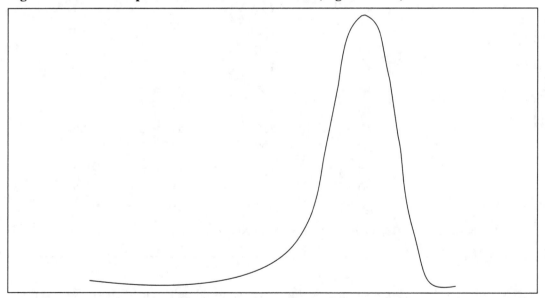

An example of skewness may occur in lengths of stay when one or more of a group of patients has an unusually long LOS. An unusually long LOS would raise the mean and thus result in a positive skewness.

Other Curves

Although less common than the normal, positive, and negative skewed curves, you may come across other types of curves in the graphical representation of data. Some examples

Figure 10.5.   **Bimodal**

Figure 10.6.   **Multimodal**

Figure 10.7.   **J-shaped**

Figure 10.8.   **Reverse J-shaped**

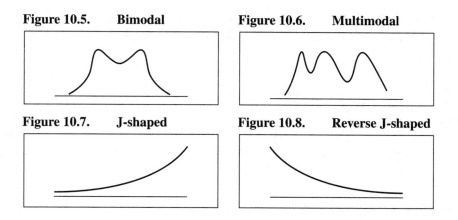

of the other types of curves include a bimodal distribution, multimodal distribution, a J-shaped curve, and a reverse J-shaped curve, which are shown in figures 10.5–10.8.

Correlation

Correlation (represented by *r*) measures the extent of a linear relationship between two variables and can be described as strong, moderate, or weak, and positive or negative. A positive relationship between two variables is direct, and a negative relationship is inverse. An example of a direct relationship is height and weight; generally the taller a person is, the more he or she weighs. An example of an inverse relationship could be when the number of prescriptions for hormone replacement therapy written by physicians goes down, the prescriptions for antidepressants goes up. It is important to remember that correlation does not imply causation; in other words, just because two variables are highly correlated does not mean that one *causes* the other.

The value for correlation will always be between –1 and +1. A correlation of 0 means there is no relationship between the variables. The closer *r* is to –1 or +1, the stronger the relationship, and the closer *r* is to 0 the weaker the relationship. –1 implies a perfect negative (inverse) relationship and +1 implies a perfect positive (direct) relationship. Chapter 11 shows three sample scatter diagrams showing a positive and negative relationship, and one showing no relationship.

To compute the correlation *r* between values *x* and *y,* use the formula:

$$r = \frac{\sum xy - \dfrac{\sum x \sum y}{n}}{\sqrt{\left(\sum x^2 - \dfrac{(\sum x)^2}{n}\right)\left(\sum y^2 - \dfrac{(\sum y)^2}{n}\right)}}$$

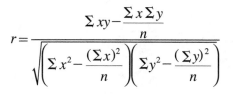

Where:

$\sum x$ is the sum of all the *x* values.

$\sum y$ is the sum of all the *y* values.

$\sum xy$ is the sum of all the *x* values multiplied by the *y* values.

$\sum x^2$ is the sum of the squares of all *x* values.

$\sum y^2$ is the sum of the squares of all *y* values.

n is the number of subjects in the group.

Example: In this example, x = the number of phone calls per week to make an appointment to see a new psychologist; y = the number of actual visits to the psychologist plus any walk-ins.

Raw Values

x	y
5	1
6	4
9	8
11	9
14	14
15	16
21	18

$$\bar{x} = 11.57 \qquad \bar{y} = 10$$
$$\Sigma x = 81 \qquad \Sigma y = 70$$
$$\Sigma x^2 = 1,125 \qquad \Sigma y^2 = 938$$
$$(\Sigma x)^2 = 6,561 \qquad (\Sigma y)^2 = 4,900$$
$$n = 7 \qquad n = 7$$
$$xy = 1,014$$

In this example, the values for Σx, Σy, Σx^2, Σy^2, $(\Sigma x)^2$, $(\Sigma y)^2$ and Σxy are computed as follows:

$\Sigma x = (5 + 6 + 9 + 11 + 14 + 15 + 21)$
$\Sigma x = 81$

$\Sigma y = (1 + 4 + 8 + 9 + 14 + 16 + 18)$
$\Sigma y = 70$

$\Sigma x^2 = (5^2 + 6^2 + 9^2 + 11^2 + 14^2 + 15^2 + 21^2)$
$\Sigma x^2 = 1,125$

$\Sigma y^2 = (1^2 + 4^2 + 8^2 + 9^2 + 14^2 + 16^2 + 18^2)$
$\Sigma y^2 = 938$

$\Sigma(x)^2 = (81)^2$
$\Sigma(x)^2 = 6,561$

$\Sigma(y)^2 = (70)^2$
$\Sigma(y)^2 = 4,900$

$\Sigma xy = (5 \times 1) + (6 \times 4) + (9 \times 8) + (11 \times 9) + (14 \times 14) + (15 \times 16) + (21 \times 18)$
$\Sigma xy = 1,014$

Next, plug these values into the formula for r.

$$r = \frac{1,014 - \dfrac{(81)(70)}{7}}{\sqrt{\left(1,125 - \dfrac{6,561}{7}\right)\left(938 - \dfrac{4,900}{7}\right)}}$$

$$r = \frac{1,014 - 810}{\sqrt{(1,125 - 937.29)(938 - 700)}}$$

$$r = \frac{204}{\sqrt{(187.71)(238)}}$$

$$r = 0.97$$

In this example, $r = 0.97$ is a very strong positive correlation. Although causation cannot be implied, it can still be said that there is a strong direct relationship between x and y. In this case, there is a very strong correlation between the number of appointments made and the number of actual visits made with the psychologist.

Calculating the correlation can be a lengthy process, especially if there are a large number of subjects. Therefore, after learning how to do the process by hand, it is best to use computer software or a calculator that is capable of computing r from keying in the values of x and y; in this way, your answer will be accurate.

Calculations for variance, standard deviation, and correlation are not usually part of the health information technician's day-to-day activities; however, it is important to be familiar with these concepts. For example, you may pick up a journal article, listen to a speaker who is discussing these calculations, or be asked to validate the data. An understanding of them may be necessary in order to communicate this information with others.

Chapter 10 Test

1. Your medical terminology instructor listed the following grades for the class out of a 75-point test:

   33, 34, 43, 45, 45, 54, 55, 59, 60, 62, 64, 66, 67, 68, 67, 68, 68, 69, 70, 70
   a. Find the 90th percentile.
   b. Your score was 59; what is your percentile?

2. From the following list of number of discharges each day in September, compute the mean, median, mode, and range. Round the mean and median to one decimal point.

Community Hospital
Number of Discharge Days
September 20XX

Day	No. of Discharges	Day	No. of Discharges	Day	No. of Discharges
1	27	11	36	21	53
2	22	12	75	22	59
3	35	13	65	23	54
4	63	14	84	24	52
5	42	15	37	25	32
6	55	16	38	26	64
7	62	17	62	27	67
8	65	18	65	28	69
9	32	19	48	29	58
10	35	20	55	30	55

(continued on next page)

Chapter 10 Test (continued)

3. Use the following dates to compute the ALOS and median LOS and range. The discharge date is July 2nd (non-leap year). Round the ALOS to one decimal place.

Admission Date	**LOS**
1-2	January = 29; February = 28; March = 31; April = 30; May = 31; June = 30; July = 2; Total = 181
1-10	January = 21; February = 28; March = 31; April = 30; May = 31; June = 30; July = 2; Total = 173
2-8	February = 20; March = 31; April = 30; May = 31; June = 30; July = 2; Total = 144
2-10	February = 18; March = 31; April = 30; May = 31; June = 30; July = 2; Total = 142
2-26	February = 2; March = 31; April = 30; May = 31; June = 30; July = 2; Total = 126
3-1	March = 30; April = 30; May = 31; June = 30; July = 2; Total = 123
3-6	March = 25; April = 30; May = 31; June = 30; July = 2; Total = 118
3-12	March = 19; April = 30; May = 31; June = 30; July = 2; Total = 112
3-15	March = 16; April = 30; May = 31; June = 30; July = 2; Total = 109
4-1	April = 29; May = 31; June = 30; July = 2; Total = 92
4-15	April = 15; May = 31; June = 30; July = 2; Total = 78
5-3	May = 28; June = 30; July = 2; Total = 60
5-5	May = 26; June = 30; July = 2; Total = 58
5-6	May = 25; June = 30; July = 2; Total = 57
5-18	May = 13; June = 30; July = 2; Total = 45
6-17	June = 13; July = 2; Total = 15
6-29	June = 1; July = 2; Total = 3
7-1	July 2; Total = 1

4. When two variables are correlated, it means that one is the cause of the other. True or false?

Chapter 10 Test (continued)

5. The table below shows the LOS for a sample of 11 discharged patients. Using the data in the table, calculate the mean, range, variance, and standard deviation, and then answer questions e and f. Round the variance and standard deviation to one decimal place.

   a. Mean
   b. Range
   c. Variance
   d. Standard deviation
   e. What value is affecting the mean and SD of this distribution?
   f. Does the mean adequately represent this distribution? If not, what would be a better measure of central tendency for this data set?

Patient	Length of Stay	LOS – Mean (5) $(X - \overline{X})$	(LOS – Mean)^2 $(X - \overline{X})^2$
1	1		
2	3		
3	5		
4	3		
5	2		
6	29		
7	3		
8	4		
9	2		
10	1		
11	2		

Chapter 11
Presentation of Data

Key Terms

Bar chart

Bar graph

Categorical data

Continuous data

Discrete data

Frequency polygon

Histogram

Interval data

Line graph

Nominal data

Ordinal data

Pictogram

Pie chart

Pie graph

Ratio data

Run chart

Scales of measurement

Scatter diagram

Table

Objectives

At the conclusion of this chapter, you should be able to:

- Discuss categorical data: nominal, ordinal, interval, and ratio

- Differentiate between discrete data and continuous data

- Describe and differentiate between tables and the following graphs: bar graphs, pie charts, line graphs, histograms, frequency polygons, pictograms, and scatter diagrams

- Create tables and graphs to display statistical information

- Understand the basic elements in preparing a report

Types of Data

A set of raw data may not necessarily provide a user (such as an administrator, a physician, or an HIM professional) with information that can be easily interpreted. Descriptive statistics are the most common type of statistics that the health information technician will encounter or be responsible for producing. Descriptive statistics describe populations, which can refer to patients, medical services, nursing units, or hospital departments. As mentioned in Chapter 10, these statistics provide an overview of the general features of a set of data. The statistics can assume a number of different forms, the most common being tables and graphs. However, before choosing the appropriate method for displaying a set of data, it is important to determine whether the data are categorical or numerical.

Categorical Data

There are four types or **scales of measurement** of **categorical data:** nominal, ordinal, ratio, and interval. Ratio and interval data are considered metric variables. Metric variables are numeric variables that answer questions of how much or how many.

Nominal Data

Nominal data are the lowest level of measurement. The word *nominal* means "pertaining to a name." In the nominal scale, observations are organized into categories in which there is no recognition of order. Examples of nominal data include true/false, male/female, types of insurance carriers, or patient occupations. Often numbers are used to represent categories. For example, a male may be listed as 1 and a female as 2; or persons may be grouped according to blood type, where 1 represents type A; 2, type B; 3, type AB; and 4, type O. The sequence of the values is not important. The numbers simply serve as labels for some piece of information and are used for convenience only.

Averages cannot be computed on nominal-level data. For example, an average blood type of 2.3 for a given population is meaningless. Instead of calculating the mean for nominal data, the proportion (or "how many") that falls into each category is reported.

The following types of healthcare payment categories are an example of nominal data.

Payment Categories
1 Medicare
2 Medicaid
3 Blue Cross
4 Other Commercial Insurance
5 Self-pay
6 Other

Ordinal Data

Ordinal data are types of data where the values are in ordered categories. The word *ordinal* means "to put something in order." On the ordinal scale, only the order of the numbers is meaningful, not the numbers themselves. This is because the intervals or distances between categories are not necessarily equal. For example, head injuries may be classified according to level of severity, where 4 is fatal; 3, severe; 2, moderate; and 1, minor.

A natural order exists among the groupings, with the largest number representing the most serious level of injury. However, the order could be reversed; there is no hard-and-fast rule. There is no reason why 1 could not represent the fatal injury and 4, the minor injury. In addition, the distance between a fatal and a severe injury may not necessarily be the same as the distance between a moderate and a minor injury. The following list shows how this works in a classification of brain injury.

1   Minor

2   Moderate

3   Severe

4   Fatal

Another good example of ordinal data is the Likert scale used in many surveys: 1 = strongly disagree; 2 = disagree; 3 = neutral; 4 = agree; 5 = strongly agree. In this example, there is a natural order 1 through 5; however, 1 could just as easily be "strongly agree" and 5, "strongly disagree."

Interval Data

Interval data include units of equal size, such as intelligence quotient (IQ) results. There is no zero point. The most important characteristic is that the intervals between values are equal. An example of interval scale is time. Time is measured in terms of 24 hours in a day. The time between each hour is the same. For example, there are 60 minutes between 1:00 a.m. and 2:00 a.m. and between 5:00 p.m. and 6:00 p.m.

Ratio Data

Ratio data or scale is the highest level of measurement. On the ratio scale, there is a defined unit of measure, a real zero point, and the intervals between successive values are equal. Ratio data may be displayed by units of equal size placed on a scale starting with zero and thus can be manipulated mathematically, such as 0, 5, 10, 15, and 20.

> **Example:** An example of the ratio scale is age. The difference between two consecutive years would be the same (the difference between age 1 and 2 is one year; the difference between age 55 and 56 is one year, and so on). There is a "zero point" in that zero would mean an absence of age or birth; and someone who is 100 years old is twice as old as someone who is 50 years old.

Exercise 11.1

Review the following table and answer the questions below.

Discharges by Gender
Annual Statistics, 20XX

Males	1,203
Females	1,235

1. What example of scales of measurement is depicted in the table?

2. Your health information instructor reported that on the last test given, 5 students received an A, 10 received a B, 3 received a C, 1 received a D, and no one received an F. What example of scales of measurement was given?

3. Is it accurate to state that a temperature of 80 degrees F is twice as hot as 40 degrees F?

4. If a physician's office saw 50 patients yesterday and 100 patients today, is it correct to state that twice as many patients were seen today as yesterday?

5. A physician's clinic conducted a survey to determine the level of patient satisfaction with various departments in the clinic. What type of scale is the following survey item?

> The information clerk at the clinic gave me the correct directions to find the department I was looking for.
>
> Please answer this question on a scale from 1 to 5 where 1 = strongly disagree and 5 = strongly agree.

6. A physician on your staff asked you to help her collect information on the effects of drinking alcohol on pregnancy and the birth weight of babies. You were asked to collect the following information.

   Did the mothers drink alcohol during pregnancy (yes or no)

   Birth weight of the baby

   Apgar score at one minute

   Apgar score at five minutes

   The scales of these variables would be:

   a. Nominal, ordinal, interval, ratio
   b. Nominal, ratio, ordinal, ordinal
   c. Ordinal, nominal, ratio, interval
   d. Ratio, ordinal, interval, nominal

Numerical Data

There are two types of numerical statistical data: discrete data and continuous data.

Discrete Data

Discrete data are finite numbers. That is, they can have only specified values. The number of children in a family is an example of discrete data. A family can have two or three children but cannot have 2.25 or 3.5 children. The numbers represent actual measurable quantities rather than labels.

Other examples of discrete data include the number of motor vehicle accidents in a particular community, the number of times a woman has given birth, the number of new cases of cancer in your state within the past five years, and the number of beds available in your hospital.

In discrete data, a natural order exists among the possible data values. In the example of the number of times a woman has given birth, a larger number indicates that she has had more children; the difference between one and two births is the same as the difference between four and five; and the number of births is restricted to whole numbers (a woman cannot give birth 2.3 times). For the most part, measurements on the nominal and ordinal scales are discrete.

Continuous Data

Continuous data represent measurable quantities but are not restricted to certain specified values. A variable that is continuous can take on a fractional value. For example, a patient's temperature may be 102.6° F. Another example is height. One could say that someone is approximately 6 feet tall, refine it to 5 feet 10 inches, and refine it still further to 5 feet $10\frac{1}{2}$ inches. Age is yet another example. You may have been 20 years old on your last birthday, but now you are 20 plus some part of another year.

The only limiting factor for a continuous observation is the degree of accuracy with which it can be measured. For analysis, continuous data often are converted to a range that acts as a category. For example, age can be categorized in ranges (0–20, 21–40, and so on). Measurements on the interval and ratio scales can be grouped; interval and ratio variables are continuous.

Data Display

Data display is critical to data analysis because it reveals patterns and behaviors. When preparing a statistical report, the user must define its objectives and scope:

- What information is needed?

- What information is available?

- Are the data collected routinely by the facility, or must additional data be collected?

If the purpose requires frequencies, percentages, or relationships among variables, the data may be presented in the form of a table or a graph. Basically, statistical tables are used for summarizing data; they simply list values into rows and columns and do not easily capture the audience's attention. On the other hand, graphs and charts can present data for quick visualization of relationships.

Tables

A **table** is an orderly arrangement of values that groups data into rows and columns. Almost any type of quantitative information can be grouped into tables. Columns allow you to read data up and down, and rows allow you to read data across. The columns and rows should be labeled. Many word-processing, spreadsheet, and database software programs offer assistance in the creation of tables. In table 11.1, variables arranged in columns across the page identify the individual patient name, age, clinical service, and length of stay. Each row represents one patient.

There are a number of advantages to using tables, including:

- More information can be presented.
- Exact values can be read to retain precision.
- Supportive details can be provided.
- Less work and fewer costs are required in the preparation.
- Flexibility is maintained without distortion of data.

The essential components of a table include:

- Title: The title must explain as simply as possible what is contained in the table. The title should answer the questions:
  — What are the data? For example, are these percentages; frequencies?

Table 11.1.   Community Medical Center analysis showing patients discharged 12/1/20XX

Name	Age	Clinical Service	Length of Stay
Smith	5	Surgical	1
Valdez	22	Obstetrical	1
Chu	26	Obstetrical	2
MacDuff	18	Obstetrical	3
Johnson	10	Surgical	7
O'Brien	80	Surgical	8
Lewandowski	35	Surgical	11
Jones	52	Medical	15
Shultz	69	Medical	37
Martini	49	Medical	42

Source: Community Medical Center.

— Who? Who is the table about? For instance, are these males or females; a certain service; a type of disease?

— Where? For example, is this your hospital; the United States; or your state?

— When? What is the time period?

- Stub heading: The title or heading of the first column
- Column headings: The headings or titles for the columns
- Stubs: The categories (the left-hand column of a table)
- Cells: The information formed by intersecting columns and rows
- Source footnote: The source for any factual data should be identified in a footnote.

Table 11.2 illustrates the essential components of a table.

Table 11.2.   The essential components of a table

	Title		
Stub Heading	**Column Heading**	**Column Heading**	**Column Heading**
Stub	Cell	Cell	Cell
Stub	Cell	Cell	Cell
Stub	Cell	Cell	Cell

Source: Reprinted, with permission, from SEER Program, Self-Instructional Manual for Cancer Registrars, Book 7 (Washington, DC: US Department of Health and Human Services, 1994, p. 23).

Table 11.3 shows a sample table with completed components.

Table 11.3.   Lung cancer by age and gender at Community Hospital, 20XX

Community Hospital Lung Cancer by Age and Gender Annual Statistics, 20XX		
Age, years	**Male**	**Female**
≤ 30	1	0
31–40	2	1
41–50	2	1
51–60	10	10
61–70	42	44
71+	29	27
Total	**86**	**83**

Although these rules are important in the construction of tables, it is more important to use good judgment. Check the table to be sure that it is logical and self-explanatory. Are headings specific and understandable for every column and row? Are sources identified, if appropriate? Do totals add up in columns and rows? Is the table easy to read? Remember to present the data in a format that illustrates a specific idea.

Frequency Distribution Tables

A frequency distribution shows the values that a variable can take and the number of observations associated with each value. A variable is a characteristic or property that may take on different values. For example, third-party payers, discharge service, and admission day are examples of variables.

> **Example:** The Utilization Review Committee is interested in knowing the admission days for patients in your hospital. To construct a frequency distribution, you would list the days of the week and then enter the observations or number of patients admitted on the corresponding day of the week. Table 11.4 illustrates what this would look like.

A frequency distribution table also may show the proportion, that is, the proportion of patients admitted on any of the days. To determine this, the value is divided by the total. The total should always equal 1.00.

Table 11.5 shows the same frequency distribution as in the example in table 11.4, but with the proportion added. Notice that to arrive at the proportion, the student should divide the number of patients admitted by the total. For example, Sunday shows 20 admissions of the 132 total.

$$\frac{20}{132} = 0.15$$

Table 11.6 shows a frequency distribution table of cigarette consumption in the United States from 1900 to 2005.

Table 11.4.   Report illustrating sample frequency distribution table

Sample Frequency Distribution for Admission Day June 20XX	
Day of the Week	**No. of Patients Admitted**
Sunday	20
Monday	29
Tuesday	28
Wednesday	12
Thursday	13
Friday	22
Saturday	8
Total	**132**

Table 11.5.   Report illustrating sample frequency distribution with proportion

Sample Frequency Distribution for Admission Day June 20XX		
Day of the Week	**No. of Patients Admitted**	**Proportion**
Sunday	20	0.15
Monday	29	0.22
Tuesday	28	0.21
Wednesday	12	0.09
Thursday	13	0.10
Friday	22	0.17
Saturday	8	0.06
Total	**132**	**1.00**

Table 11.6.   Report illustrating frequency distribution

Cigarette Consumption, United States, 1900–2005	
Year	**No. of Cigarettes Consumed (in billions)**
1900	2.5
1905	3.6
1910	8.6
1915	17.9
1920	44.6
1925	79.8
1930	119.3
1935	134.4
1940	181.9
1945	340.6
1950	369.8
1955	396.4
1960	484.4
1965	528.8
1970	536.5
1975	607.2
1980	631.5
1985	594.0
1990	525.0
1995	487.0
2000	430.0
2005	376.0

Source: Tobacco Outlook Report, Economic Research Service, US Dept. of Agriculture. Available at http://www.infoplease.com/ipa/A0908700.html.

To display discrete or continuous data in the form of a frequency distribution table, the range of values of the observations must be broken down into a series of distinct groups that do not overlap. For example, when arranging a frequency distribution table by patient age, age ranges should not be listed as 1–10, 10–20, 20–30, 30–40, and so on because a patient could be placed in two categories if he were age 20: the 10 to 20 age range and the 20 to 30 age range. Thus, age ranges should be listed as 1–10, 11–20, 21–30, 31–40, and so on.

Summarizing the data involves setting up categories and counting the number of cases that fall into each category, thereby creating a frequency distribution. Following are some general rules for choosing the classes or categories into which the data are to be grouped and the range of each:

- Do not use fewer than five or more than 15 categories. However, the choice depends mostly on the number of values to be grouped.

- Categories should be well defined. Choose categories that cover the smallest and largest values and do not produce gaps between categories.

- The categories should be mutually exclusive where each observation is grouped into one—and only one—category. Avoid successive classes that overlap or have common values.

- Whenever possible, make the classes cover equal ranges (or intervals) of values. These ranges also should be made up of numbers that are easy to work with.

Exercise 11.2

The table below lists the patients seen last month at Community Hospital with their age and cholesterol reading. Create a table using common age categories and these ranges for cholesterol:

Desirable ≤ 199
Borderline High 200–239
High ≥ 240

Age	Cholesterol	Age	Cholesterol	Age	Cholesterol	Age	Cholesterol
14	118	44	138	38	165	56	185
80	139	47	204	18	142	20	200
42	187	48	236	62	139	45	241
37	201	25	186	37	202	63	175
23	107	56	201	32	207	70	188
24	109	47	198	17	157	42	239
67	132	20	210	55	238	55	175
55	235	43	248	13	134	61	168
52	185	50	137	44	239	53	173
52	192	34	188	64	165	41	238
47	144	38	245	70	172	60	180
42	158	75	175	44	245	30	207
37	160	55	207	65	187	62	185
33	155	69	192	51	248	49	207
39	221	31	196	43	240	39	147
34	244	51	147	51	188	53	155
75	186	63	200	50	203	46	246
81	160	18	137	20	145	43	222
79	154	37	245	72	175	26	147
67	154	43	256	39	200	46	201
50	192	44	188	19	145	60	152
53	188	52	200	63	145	35	150
26	137	51	147	36	176	53	215
24	140	19	132	33	185	60	165
22	138	73	147	16	137	63	168

Exercise 11.3

The following table shows a frequency distribution of patients with colon cancer treated at Community Hospital. Compute the proportion of patients in each category.

Community Hospital
Ages of Patients with Colon Cancer
Annual Statistics, 20XX

Age	No. of Patients	Proportion
≤ 30	3	
31–40	12	
41–50	18	
51–60	60	
61–70	65	
71+	48	

Graphs

Graphs of various types are the best means for presenting data for quick visualization of relationships. They often supply a lesser degree of detail than tables. However, data presented in a graph can be helpful in displaying statistics in a concise manner. There are advantages to using graphs. They grab the audience's attention and are easy to understand. They can show trends or comparisons.

Graphs should be easy to read, simple in content, and correctly labeled. The presentation of data in the form of a graph is an excellent way to convey the message you want to get across. Instead of presenting an entire statistical report in a table to a group such as the medical staff or administration, you can create a graph to depict the data. Many computer software programs are available that convert data into graphic form automatically and attractively.

When creating graphs, follow these general guidelines:

- The title must relate to what the graph is displaying. Follow the same general guidelines for the title in graphs as given in tables including what are the data, what is the graph about, to whom does it refer, and the time period.

- When several variables are included on the same graph (for example, males and females), each should be identified by using a legend or key.

- Categories should be natural; that is, the vertical axis should always start with zero. The scale of values for the x-axis reads from the lowest value on the left to the highest on the right. The scale of values for the y-axis extends from the lowest value at the bottom of the graph to the highest at the top.

- Scale captions are placed on both axes to identify the values clearly. These are simply titles placed on each axis to identify the values. (See figure 11.1.)

Figure 11.1.   Scale captions on a graph

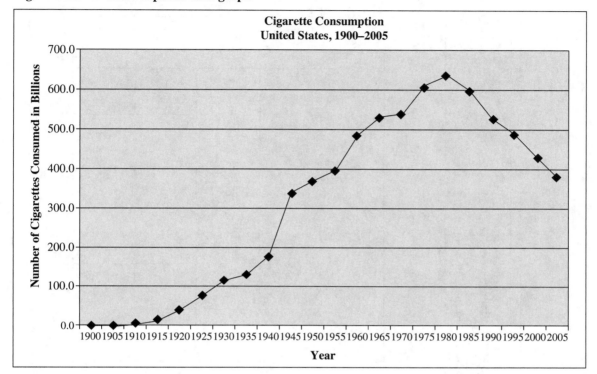

- Graphs should emphasize the horizontal. It is easier for the eye to read along the horizontal axis from left to right. Also, graphs should be greater in length than in height. A useful guideline is to follow the three-quarter-high rule, which states that the graph's height (y-axis) should be three-fourths of its length (x-axis).

- The exact reference to an outside source should be given.

Handy Tip: Selecting the most appropriate graph to accompany your data adds a great deal to the effectiveness of your presentation; however, you should avoid an overabundance of graphs. It is a good idea to produce several versions of a graph and then use the one that is most illuminating (SEER Program 1994).

Bar Graphs

Bar graphs, or **bar charts,** are appropriate for displaying categorical data. The simplest bar graph is a one-variable bar graph. In this type of graph, the various categories of observations are presented along a horizontal axis, or x-axis. (See figures 11.2 and 11.3.) The vertical axis, or y-axis, displays the frequency of the data. Data representing frequencies, proportions, or percentages of categories are often displayed using bar graphs. A grouped bar chart is used to display information from tables containing two or three variables. Figure 11.4 shows an example of a three-variable bar graph.

Figure 11.2.   Example of a one-variable bar graph

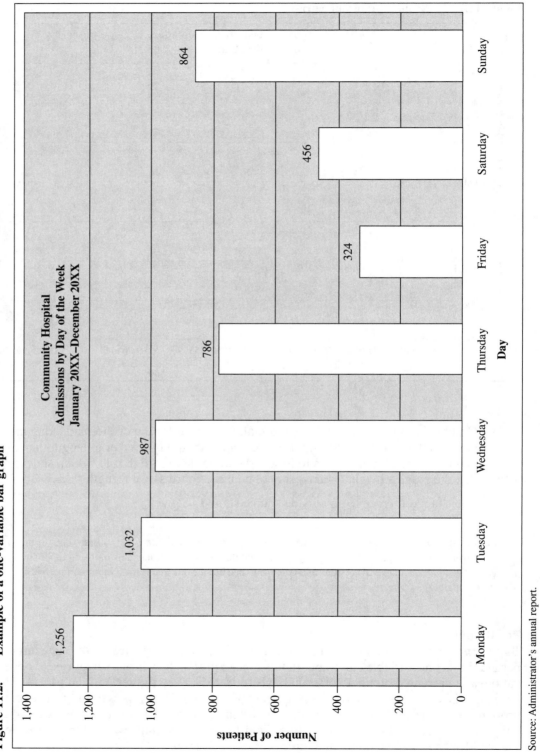

Community Hospital
Admissions by Day of the Week
January 20XX–December 20XX

Source: Administrator's annual report.

Figure 11.3.   **Example of a two-variable bar graph**

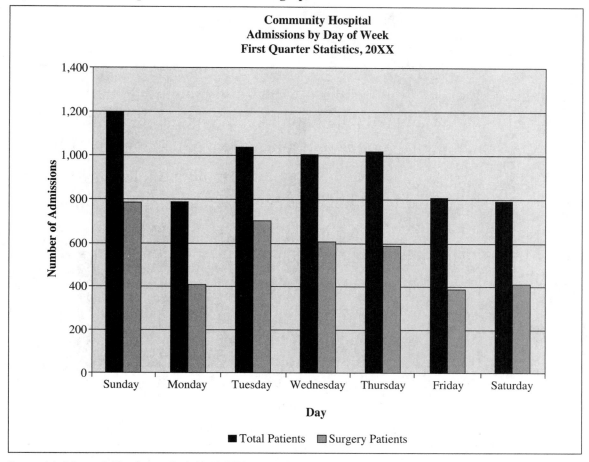

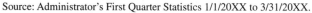

Source: Administrator's First Quarter Statistics 1/1/20XX to 3/31/20XX.

Figure 11.4.   Example of a three-variable bar graph

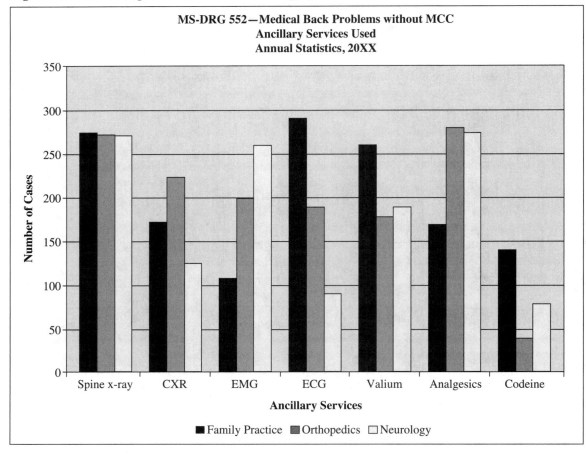

Pie Charts

A **pie chart,** or **pie graph,** is a method of displaying data as component parts of a whole. It is an easily understood chart in which the sizes of the slices of the pie show the proportional contribution of each part. Use a pie chart when you want to show each category's percentage of the total. A circle is divided into sections such as wedges or slices. These represent percentages of the total (100 percent). To make a pie chart, include all the categories that make up a whole. Therefore, data must be converted into percentages unless you are working with computer software that converts your numbers into percentages. Pie chart wedges may be shaded or colored to help differentiate the sections. In addition, they can be cut out of the pie to help emphasize a percentage. Computer software programs are extremely useful when creating pie graphs. (See figures 11.5 and 11.6 for examples of pie charts.)

Figure 11.5.   Pie graph showing nosocomial infection by major service category

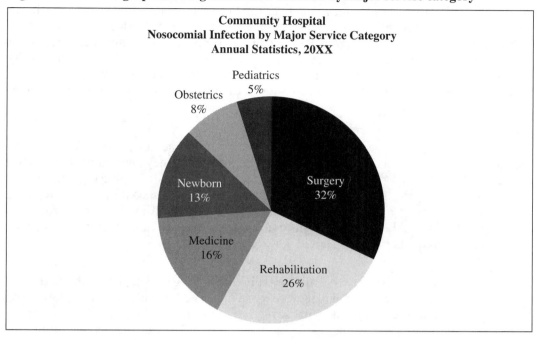

Community Hospital
Nosocomial Infection by Major Service Category
Annual Statistics, 20XX

Figure 11.6.   Pie graph showing brain injury patients admitted from other facilities

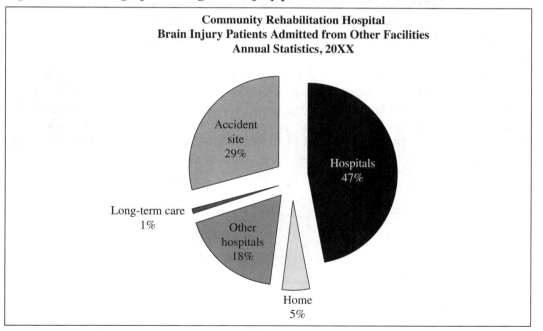

Community Rehabilitation Hospital
Brain Injury Patients Admitted from Other Facilities
Annual Statistics, 20XX

Line Graphs

A **line graph** is often used to show data over time (for example, days, weeks, months, or years). The x-axis shows the time period, and the y-axis shows the values of the variables. A line graph consists of a line connecting a series of points. Line graphs also allow for several variables to be plotted. Line graphs are also referred to as **run charts** in the quality management field. The x-axis depicts the units of time from left to right, and the y-axis measures the values of the variable being shown. (See figures 11.7 and 11.8 for examples of line graphs.)

Histograms

A **histogram** is a graph used to display frequency distributions for continuous numerical data (interval or ratio data). Histograms are created from frequency distribution tables. (See figures 11.9 and 11.10 for examples of histograms.) They look similar to bar graphs except that all the bars in a histogram are touching because they show the continuous nature of the distribution. In histograms the bars should be of equal width. Ordinarily in constructing a histogram, there should not be less than four and usually never more than twelve bars or classes and the frequency groups should not overlap.

Frequency Polygon

A **frequency polygon** is similar to a histogram in that it is a graph depicting the frequency of continuous data; however, a frequency polygon is in line form instead of bar form. The advantage of a frequency polygon is that several of them can be placed on the same graph to make comparisons. A frequency polygon uses the same axes as the histogram; that is, the x-axis displays the scale of the variable and the y-axis displays the frequency. A dot is placed at the midpoint of the class interval or frequency. A line drawn from one point to the next then connects the dots. Because the x-axis represents the entire frequency distribution, the line starts at zero cases and is drawn from the last frequency to the y-axis to end with zero. (See figure 11.11.)

Pictogram

A **pictogram** is an attractive alternative type of bar graph in that it uses pictures to show the frequency of the data. For example, if you want to show the top five cancer site deaths, you might use stick people. If you need to show exact numbers, a pictogram will probably not be a good choice for your presentation; however, they are very good at catching the attention of your audience and will give them a good sense of your data. (See figure 11.12.)

Figure 11.7.   Example of a one-variable line graph

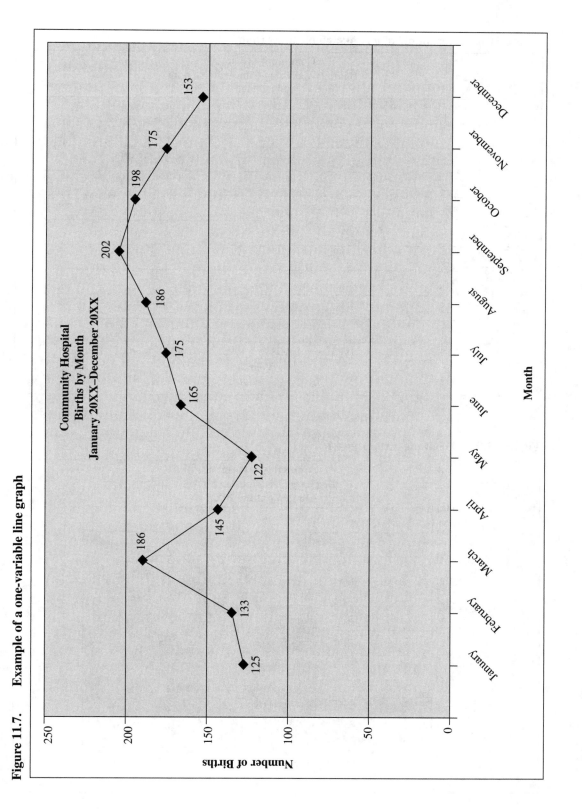

**Community Hospital
Births by Month
January 20XX–December 20XX**

Figure 11.8.   Example of a two-variable line graph

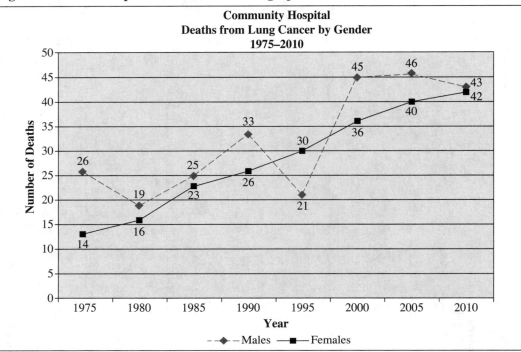

Figure 11.9.   Sample histogram #1

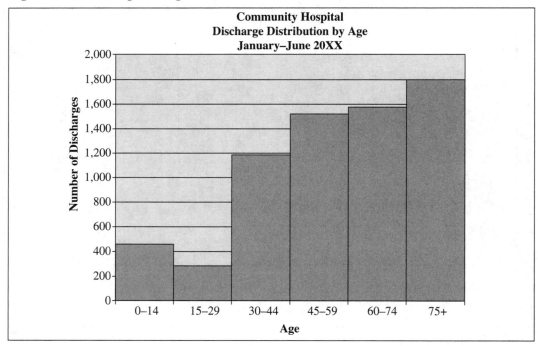

Figure 11.10.   Sample histogram #2

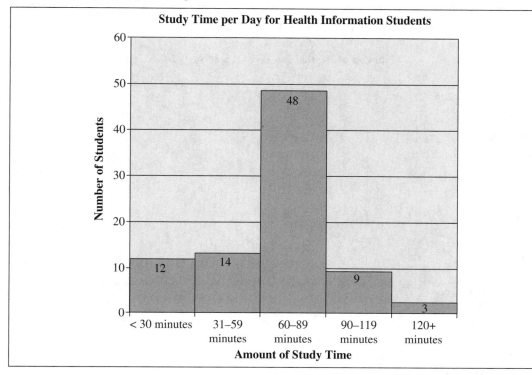

Figure 11.11.   Frequency polygon

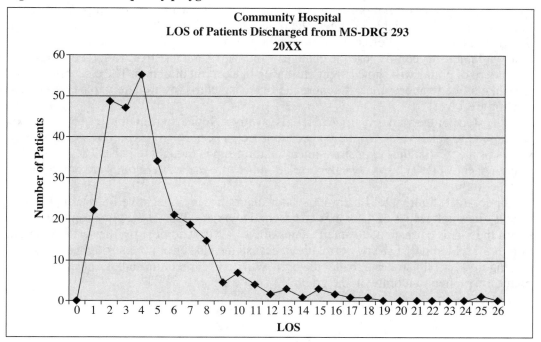

Figure 11.12.   Sample pictogram

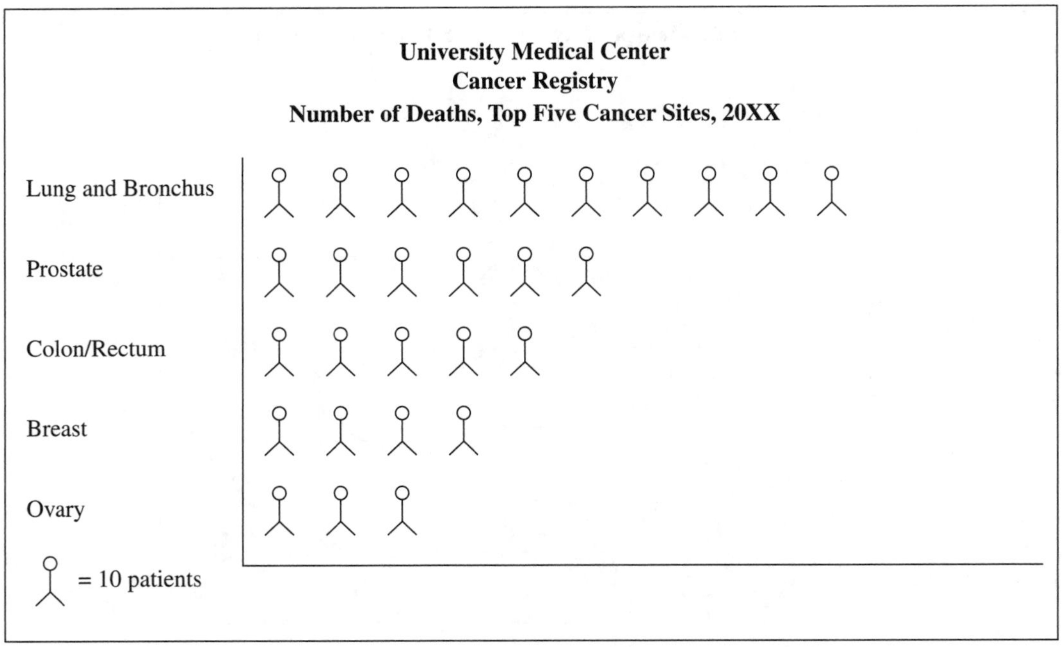

Scatter Diagram

A **scatter diagram** (also called a scattergram or scatter plot) is used to graphically show the relationship between two numerical variables. A scatter diagram is used to determine whether there is a correlation, or relationship, between two characteristics. Correlation implies that as one variable changes, the other also changes. This does not always mean that there is a cause-and-effect relationship between two variables because there may be other variables that could cause the change. If the two characteristics are somehow related, the pattern of points will show a tight clustering in a certain direction. The closer the points look like a line in appearance, the more the two characteristics are likely to be correlated. (See figure 11.13.)

The slope of the values in figure 11.13 is positive. Notice that small values of the x-axis correspond to small values of the y-axis and large values of the x-axis correspond to large values of the y-axis; thus, a positive linear relationship is thought to exist. The scatter diagram in figure 11.13 shows a weak correlation because the scatter points are not clustered together tightly.

In contrast, figure 11.14 shows a scatter diagram with a negative linear relationship. That is, the small values of the x-axis correspond to large values of the y-axis and large values of the x-axis correspond to small values of the y-axis. Additionally, the scatter diagram in figure 11.14 shows a strong correlation because the cluster of points is tight.

Figure 11.15 illustrates a scatter diagram with no linear relationship because the scatter points are plotted randomly on the graph.

Figure 11.13.   Sample scatter diagram showing a positive linear relationship

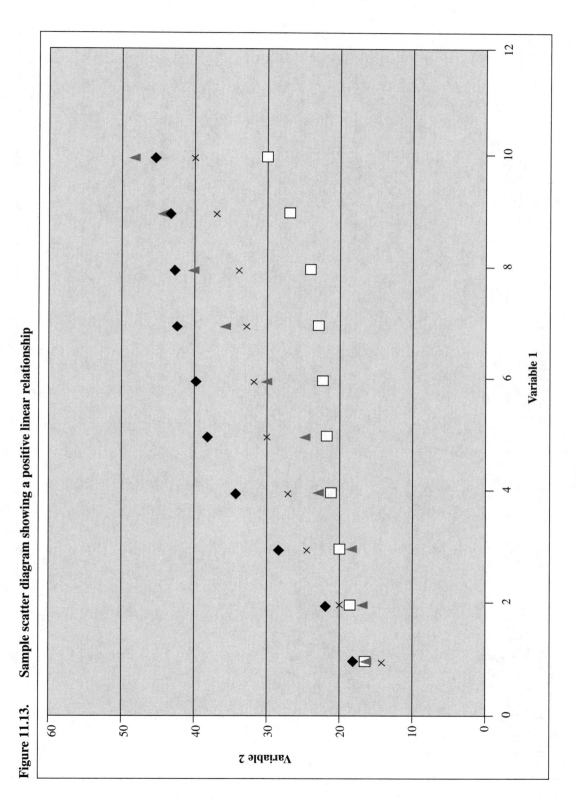

Figure 11.14.   Sample scatter diagram showing a negative linear relationship

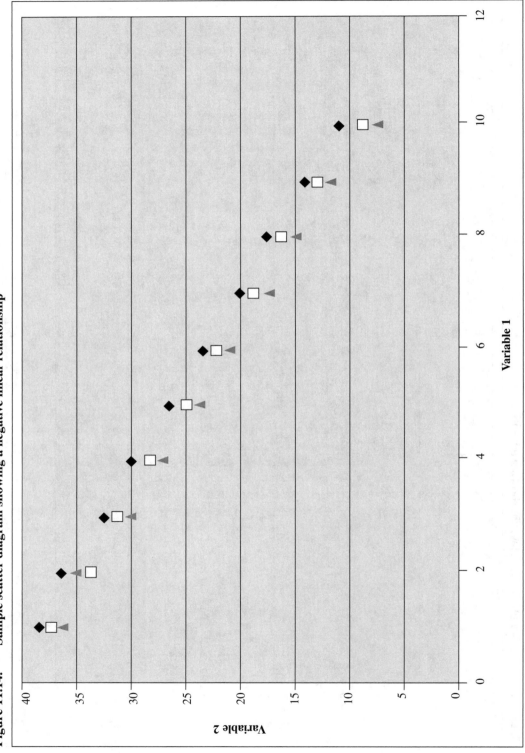

Figure 11.15.   **Sample scatter diagram showing no linear relationship**

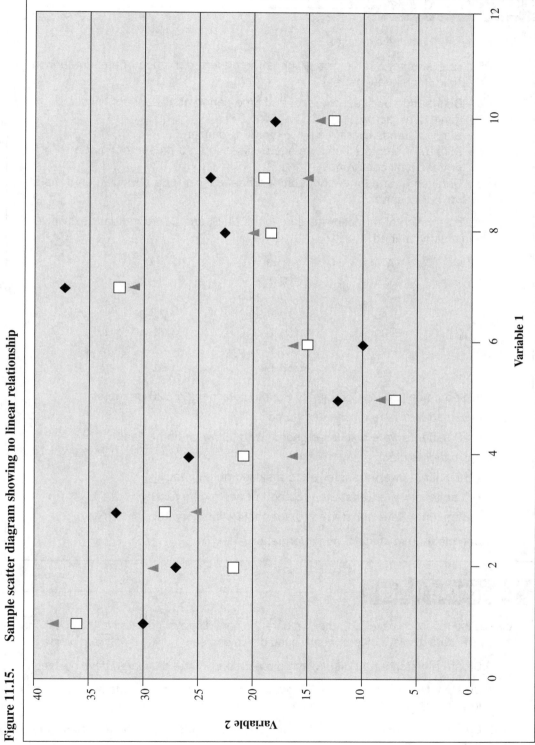

Variable 1

Variable 2

Exercise 11.4

Complete the following exercises.

1. Indicate whether a table or a graph is the preferred method of presentation in the following situations:

    a. Distribution by site, sex, race, and time period of all cancers in your healthcare facility
    b. Survival trends over time by sex for lung cancer
    c. Display of prostate cancer stage of disease for a presentation at a professional conference
    d. Detailed treatment distribution of breast cancer for a physician on the staff of your hospital

2. Indicate which of the following categories (A, B, and C) are mutually exclusive and clearly defined.

A	B	C
0–15	≤ 10.0	0–10
15–30	10.1–20.0	11–20
30–45	20.1–30.0	21–30
45–60	30.1–40.0	31–40
60+	40.1–50.0	41–50
	50.1+	51+

3. In September 2011, Community Hospital discharged 120 patients.
    - 82 patients were discharged home
    - 10 patients were discharged home with follow-up home health
    - 6 patients died
    - 11 patients were transferred to a skilled nursing facility
    - 3 patients were transferred to another acute care facility
    - 8 patients were transferred to a rehabilitation hospital

    Complete a pie chart of this information.

Exercise 11.5

Analyze the report on page 221, then prepare the data displays indicated in the questions below. The data displays may be neatly hand drawn or created using a software program.

1. Create a histogram to display the distribution of total discharge days by age.

2. Create a bar graph to display the admission by day of week for Medicare patients in comparison to the admission by day of week for all patients.

3. Create a pie chart to display the percentage of patients discharged by major service category.

4. Create a table for length of stay distribution.

Exercise 11.5 (continued)

Administrator's Semiannual Reference Report
January–June 20XX

ALL PATIENTS, INCLUDING ONE-DAY STAYS (SEPARATE)

	ADMISSIONS				DISCHARGES			
	TOTAL PTS.	% OF PTS.	SURG. PTS.	AVG. PREOP	ONE-DAY STAYS	TOTAL PTS.	% OF PTS.	AVG. LOS	ONE-DAY STAYS
SUNDAY	1,187	17.9	774	1.7	146	809	12.1	8.1	46
MONDAY	755	11.3	426	2.8	124	576	8.7	6.2	144
TUESDAY	1,085	16.3	689	2.6	135	934	14.0	7.2	115
WEDNESDAY	1,035	15.5	622	3.5	141	934	14.0	7.7	147
THURSDAY	1,024	15.3	597	2.6	139	955	14.3	7.0	132
FRIDAY	808	12.1	359	3.9	145	965	14.5	7.7	141
SATURDAY	773	11.6	417	3.0	39	1,490	22.4	6.6	144

LENGTH OF STAY DISTRIBUTION

	TOTAL PTS.	% CASES
SAME DAY	114	1.7
1 DAY	755	11.3
2–4 DAYS	1,343	20.2
5–7 DAYS	1,555	23.3
8–14 DAYS	1,469	22.0
15–42 DAYS	1,217	18.3
43+ DAYS	210	3.2

SUMMARY BY MAJOR SERVICE CATEGORY

	TOTAL PTS.	% OF PTS.	DIS DAYS	% DAYS	ALOS
MEDICINE	2,005	30.0	21,052	30.6	10.5
SURGERY	1,401	21.0	7,845	11.4	5.6
GYNECOLOGY	631	9.4	6,057	8.8	9.6
OBSTETRICS	530	7.9	2,703	3.9	5.1
NEWBORN	520	7.8	2,600	3.7	5.0
PEDIATRICS	450	6.7	4,140	6.0	9.2
PSYCHIATRY	518	7.7	8,537	12.4	16.5
OTHER	608	9.1	15,798	22.9	26.0

ADMISSION BY DAY OF THE WEEK BY PAYMENT STATUS

	SELF	BLUE CROSS	COMMERCIAL	GOV'T	WORK COMP	M-CAID	M-CARE	OTHER	TOTAL
SUNDAY	31	413	188	0	2	41	273	2	950
MONDAY	19	300	103	0	11	46	280	1	760
TUESDAY	21	400	206	1	9	45	345	2	1,029
WEDNESDAY	20	503	240	2	22	35	223	3	1,048
THURSDAY	30	365	154	0	8	24	199	1	781
FRIDAY	28	40	179	0	0	42	294	0	583
SATURDAY	30	509	246	1	6	55	301	2	1,150
TOTAL PTS.	179	2,892	1,316	4	58	288	1,915	11	
% OF PTS.	2.6	43.4	19.7	0.6	0.8	4.3	28.7	0	
TOT DIS DAYS	1,109	26,895	16,818	36	609	2,670	20,491	104	
% OF DAYS	1.6	39.1	24.4	0	0.8	4	30	0	
AVG. LOS	6.2	9.3	12.8	9.0	10.5	9.3	11	9.5	

(continued on next page)

Exercise 11.5 (continued)

SUMMARY BY AGE

	TOTAL PTS.	% OF PTS.	TOT DIS DAYS	% DAYS	ALOS
0–14	429	6.4	1,749	2.5	4.1
15–18	229	3.4	817	1.2	3.6
19–34	1,144	17.2	9,746	14.2	8.5
35–49	1,488	22.3	14,647	21.3	9.8
50–64	1,570	23.6	18,101	26.3	11.5
65+	1,803	27.1	23,672	34.4	13.1
TOTAL	**6,663**		**68,732**		**10.3**

Exercise 11.6

University Hospital Cancer Registry records show the following incidence of cancer in females for the past year. Construct an appropriate graph of the data.

University Hospital
Cancer Registry
10 Most Prevalent Cancer Sites—Females
20XX

Site	Number of Cases
Breast	120
Colon and rectum	42
Uterus	25
Thyroid	21
Lymphoma	20
Melanoma	19
Lung and bronchus	15
Ovary	12
Pancreas	8
Leukemia	6

Exercise 11.7

University Hospital reported the following incidence of lung and bronchus cancer patients treated at the hospital during the past 15 years. Construct a line graph of the data.

**University Hospital
Cancer Registry Data
Lung and Bronchus Cancer
by Year and Gender**

Year	Males	Females
1994	112	48
1995	121	47
1996	130	49
1997	123	50
1998	121	54
1999	131	55
2000	150	60
2001	155	65
2002	173	72
2003	171	75
2004	172	80
2005	171	83
2006	170	87
2007	168	93
2008	165	120
2009	169	118
2010	175	121
2011	172	120

Preparing Reports

Writing reports for your workplace is not the same as writing an article for a professional journal or preparing a report for an assignment in one of your classes, but the goal is the same. Communication is the goal and it is achieved when you write your report in the style your audience prefers. Often your healthcare administration will let you know how reports are prepared and presented in your facility, or you could review previous reports that have been given to committees or your administration to use as a guide. Some reports are more formal than others. For example, for a committee meeting you may just provide some data in the form of graphs or tables to share with the members, whereas for a Cancer Conference, where information may be shared with the community, a more formal report will be in order.

Here are some general guidelines to follow:

- Include a title for the report.
- For formal reports or one with many graphs and tables, include a table of contents.
- Include the tables and graphs.
    - Tables and graphs are great tools for presenting data. Tables show summarized and more detailed data and graphs are useful for presenting relationships in visual form. The question of which to use depends on the audience.
    - Take a few minutes before you prepare a report to think about who will be reading or seeing your presentation. Will you be presenting information to your administrator about the need for new equipment in your department; will it be to a team who is deciding whether or not to investigate the need for a new service in your facility; or will it be to a committee evaluating the quality of care provided in your hospital? Determine what you are trying to say to this person or group. Determine what details must be included, then decide what types of tables and/or graphs you want to provide.
    - Tables have several advantages over graphs:
        - More information can be presented in a table.
        - Exact values in tables can be helpful.
        - Ordinarily less work is involved in creating a table.
    - Graphs, on the other hand, also have advantages:
        - Graphs are more attention-grabbing than tables.
        - Graphs show trends more clearly.
        - Graphs bring out facts that will stimulate thinking.
- Prepare a narrative report if you are asked to provide one or if it will make the presentation more understandable.
    - Tables and graphs are just a part of the decision-making process. Adding narrative discussions to reports helps people better understand the data.
    - Narrative description can explain what the values mean.
    - Narrative reports can include historical information, for instance, what the data has shown over a specific period of time.
    - The narrative can include factors that may influence the data such as seasonal changes in the patient population or reasons for significant increases or decreases in the data.
    - Make sure your data are correct because inaccurate data may lead to inaccurate decisions.
    - Be sure to include the sources of the data.

- Write to the style of your workplace.

  — Be objective. Report all the pertinent information, both positive and negative points.

  — Use bias-free language. Avoid words such as "awesome" or "incredible."

  — Write in an impersonal style. Do not start your sentences with "I compared . . .", but rather, "A comparison showed . . ."

  — Be concise and strive for clarity.

  — Proofread your document; brush up on your grammatical skills.

Chapter 11 Test

Complete the following exercises.

1. What is one of the simplest types of categorical data where the values fall into unordered categories?

   a. Ordinal
   b. Nominal
   c. Ratio
   d. Interval

2. A graphic display can help healthcare professionals understand data. True or false?

3. What type of numerical data contains only a finite number of results?

   a. Continuous
   b. Discrete

4. In creating a frequency distribution table, which of the following statements is not a basic rule to follow?

   a. Choose classes that cover the smallest and largest values.
   b. Make certain that each item can go into only one class.
   c. As a general rule, use between 10 and 15 classes.
   d. Do not produce gaps between classes.

5. Line graphs can be used to illustrate the relationship between continuous quantities. True or false?

6. When creating histograms, which is a true statement?

   a. Form classes of equal width.
   b. Always form frequency groups that do not overlap.
   c. Establish between five and 15 frequency groups.
   d. All of the above

(continued on next page)

Chapter 11 Test (continued)

7. Which graph displays vertical bars to depict frequency distributions for continuous data?

    a. Histogram
    b. Line graph
    c. Pie graph
    d. Frequency distribution table

8. Bar graphs are used to display comparisons between nominal data. True or false?

9. What do the wedges or divisions in a pie graph represent?

    a. Frequency groups
    b. Various data
    c. Percentages
    d. Classes

10. Which of the following graphs would be best to use to display the percentages of diagnoses seen at your mental health center?

    a. Frequency polygon
    b. Pie graph
    c. Bar graph
    d. Line graph

11. Which of the following graphs would be best for the cancer registrar to use to display the five-year survival rates of lung cancer patients in the years 20XX to 20XX at your hospital?

    a. Frequency polygon
    b. Bar graph
    c. Line graph
    d. Histogram

12. Which of the following graphs would be best to use to display the number of discharges by medical service for the past year?

    a. Line graph
    b. Bar graph
    c. Histogram
    d. Frequency polygon

Chapter 12
Basic Research Principles

Key Terms

Alternative hypothesis

Applied research

Basic research

Bed size

Causal research

Cluster sampling

Conclusive research

Convenience sampling

Correlational research

Data collection

Descriptive research

Ethnography

Evaluation research

Experimental research

Exploratory research

Historical research

Hypothesis

Individually identifiable health information

Institutional Review Board

Instrument

Judgment sampling

Literature review

Naturalistic observation

Null hypothesis

Observation

Primary research

Qualitative research

Quantitative research

Questionnaire

Quota sampling

Reliability

Sample

Sample size

Secondary research

Stratified random sampling

Structured interview

Survey

Systematic random sampling

Unrestricted question

Validity

Objectives

At the conclusion of this chapter, you should be able to:

- Explain the different types of research
- Describe the difference between quantitative and qualitative research
- Differentiate among research designs: exploratory, historical, descriptive, causal, correlational, evaluation, and experimental
- Describe the steps in the research process
- Explain exploratory and conclusive research design methods
- Describe the various data-collection techniques
- Differentiate among the following types of samples: probability and nonprobability, simple random, stratified, cluster, judgment, quota, and convenience
- Define Institutional Review Board (IRB) and understand its role in research
- Define hypothesis
- Define reliability and validity
- Differentiate between primary and secondary research
- Describe the Institutional Review Board in healthcare facilities conducting research
- Understand the various data interpretation issues and the importance of verification of data
- Apply ethical guidelines in the use of statistics

Basic Research Principles

Research is the search toward the solution of problems. It answers questions that you or others may have and calls attention to theories that may be helpful in predicting future experiences.

Research is done in many fields and may be done in a variety of ways. Health research covers the wide gamut of laboratory research, clinical trials, and public health issues. This chapter covers the basic types of research and the steps in the research process, including data-collection techniques and the different types of samples.

Two Types of Research

There are generally two types of research: basic and applied. In **basic research,** the investigator is not concerned with the immediate applicability of his or her results but, rather, tries to look for understanding of natural processes. In **applied research,** the investigator has some kind of application in mind and wants to discover information about it that can be used to solve a problem or in some way contribute to society.

Research Methodology

Research methodology is the study of different types of research methods. At a higher and more general level, researchers in research methodology have described two overarching approaches to research: the qualitative approach and the quantitative approach.

Table 12.1.   Characteristics of quantitative and qualitative research

Quantitative Research	Qualitative Research
• Uses quantitative methods, including observations, experiments, and surveys	• Describes observations without the use of numerical data, including interviews, observations, and written documents
• Is objective	• Is subjective
• Uses controlled measurements	• Uses uncontrolled observations
• Researcher is removed from the data; is an outside observer	• Researcher is close to the data; has an inside perspective
• Can be generalized and replicated	• Is not generalized and may not be replicable
• Is outcome oriented	• Is process oriented

Qualitative Research

Qualitative research describes events, persons, and so on without the use of numerical data. An example of qualitative research would be interviews with health information practitioners to determine whether their past healthcare experiences affected their decision to enter the health information field or interviews with mothers of handicapped infants to determine how their lives were affected by the birth of their children. Qualitative research consists of interviews, observations, and written documents that may be used individually or in combination. "The richness of data permits a fuller understanding of what is being studied than could be derived from experimental research methods" (Best and Kahn 1993, 186).

Quantitative Research

Quantitative research uses quantitative methods, or numbers, to describe a study, including some comparisons of the population and statistical analysis to describe the results. Quantitative research consists of observations, experiments, and **surveys.**

Table 12.1 illustrates some characteristics of quantitative and qualitative research.

The Research Process

Although there are as many descriptions of the types of research as there are textbooks and articles about the subject, most agree that the research process involves the following six major steps:

1. Define the problem.

2. Review the literature.

3. Design the research.

4. Collect the data.

5. Analyze the data.

6. Draw conclusions.

Defining the Problem

Problem definition refers to forming a question regarding a topic you would like to study. The most important thing is to be clear about what you want to study. Often an analysis of historical data, or secondary information, has gone into the problem definition.

Historical data analysis simply means looking at the past to see what has been done before; it prevents reinventing the wheel. In previous research, an investigator may have made recommendations for future studies. In addition, problems may be broken down into subcomponents or smaller problems. Figure 12.1 demonstrates an example of a problem and its possible subcomponents.

The definition also may define the scope of the study, that is, who or what will be included in the study. For example, a study that includes hospitals may be defined as including only those hospitals with fewer than 100 beds, a study that involves patients may include only those patients who are age 60 and over, or a study may include females only.

Reviewing the Literature

A **literature review** is an investigation of all the information about a topic. It is important to start any study with a review of literature on the research you want to conduct for three important reasons:

1. to determine whether research has already been done on the question

2. to determine whether any data sources can be used in the study

3. to help make the hypothesis more specific

There are many sources of previous research. These may include journals, books, position papers, conference presentations, videos, interviews, and online databases, to name just a few.

Figure 12.1.   Example of a research problem and its subcomponents

Problem/Question: Should a physician clinic in your community put an organized health information department into operation?

- Subcomponent 1. What are the health information services that could be provided?
- Subcomponent 2. What types of employees should be employed in this department?
- Subcomponent 3. What amount of space is needed for the department?
- Subcomponent 4. Where should the health information department be located?
- Subcomponent 5. What equipment does the department need to be operational?
- Subcomponent 6. What would be the total estimated cost of the project?

Designing the Research and Collecting the Data

There are several types of research design, including the following:

- **Exploratory research** is often undertaken when a problem is not very clearly defined. This type of research allows the researcher to study a problem and gather information. It may generate a hypothesis. Exploratory research is generally informal and relies on literature review and informal discussions with others to find out more about a problem. Although exploratory research may not help answer the problem, it may provide insights into the problem.

- **Historical research** involves an investigation and analysis of past events. This type of research also allows the researcher to apply previous researchers' experiences and conclusions in his or her professional practice.

- **Conclusive research** is performed in order to reach some sort of conclusion or to help in decision making. This type of research may be done using **primary research,** that is, data collected specifically for your study; or **secondary research,** that is, a literature review to see if previous studies can be used to answer your question. Secondary research may also include summaries of past works. There are two types of conclusive research:

  — **Descriptive research,** or statistical research, provides data about the population you are studying, including the frequency that something occurs. These data might include studies on the status of the composition of the HIM workforce, employee morale in departments, coding accuracy, or the extent of electronic health record (EHR) implementation. The two most common collection techniques for descriptive research are observations and surveys.

  — **Causal research** tries to answer questions about what causes certain things to occur. This type of research is difficult because there may always be an additional cause to consider. Causal research uses experimentation and simulation as its data-collection methods.

- **Correlational research** refers to studies that try to discover a relationship between variables. A variable is anything under study. In correlational research, the strength of the relationship is measured and there may be a positive or a negative relationship between variables. Correlational research only determines if there is a relationship between two or more variables, it does not determine the cause of those relationships. If a strong relationship is found, experimental research can be carried out to determine causality. (See chapter 11 for a more detailed discussion on correlation.) This type of research uses **questionnaires,** observations, and secondary data as its data-collection methods. Examples of correlational research might include studying whether there is a relationship between watching violence on television and behavior, whether graduating with a 4.0 grade point average from college affects the type of job a student gets after graduation, or whether there is a relationship between eating eggs and cholesterol levels.

- **Evaluation research** is a process used to determine what has happened during a given activity or in an institution. The purpose of evaluation research is to lead to a better understanding of whether a program is effective, whether a policy is working, or whether something that was agreed upon is the most cost-effective way of doing something. For example, evaluation research may be done each year to determine whether your school's health information program is meeting its goals.

- **Experimental research** entails manipulation of a situation in some way in order to test a hypothesis. In experimental research, certain variables are kept constant and an independent or experimental variable is manipulated. Researchers select both independent and dependent variables. Independent variables are the factors that researchers manipulate directly; dependent variables are the measured variables. Examples of experimental research include studies such as determining whether a certain medication is effective in treating Parkinsonism or studying whether the use of robotic technology in the operating suite is more beneficial to patients than the traditional surgical approach.

Statement of the Hypothesis

In formal research, a **hypothesis** is formed. A hypothesis is a statement of the predicted relationship of what the researcher is studying. It is a proposed solution or explanation the researcher has reached through the literature review. More simply stated, it is the tentative answer to the question being studied.

The statement of the hypothesis is important because it allows the researcher to think about the variables and type of research design to use in the study. The research tests the hypothesis, proving it to be positive or negative (correct or incorrect). The fact that a hypothesis is rejected (that is, proven incorrect) does not necessarily mean that the research is poor but, rather, only that the results are different from what was expected. The formulation of the hypothesis in advance of the data-gathering process is necessary for an unbiased investigation.

There are two forms of the hypothesis:

- The **null hypothesis** states that there is no difference between the population means or proportions being compared or that there is no association between the two variables being compared. For example, in a clinical trial of a new medication, the null hypothesis is: The new medication is no better than the current medication. A detailed discussion of the null hypothesis is given in chapter 13.

- The **alternative hypothesis** is a statement of what the study is set up to establish. For example, in the clinical trial of a new medication, the alternative hypothesis is: The new medication is better than the current medication.

Data-Collection Techniques

Data collection includes primary research, or the data obtained from observations, surveys, and interviews. It also includes secondary research, or the literature review or summaries of original studies. Regardless of the data-collection method used, the research must be valid and reliable.

- **Validity** is the degree to which scientific observations actually measure or record what they purport to measure. For example, if the researcher is using a written questionnaire to collect data, he or she will pretest it by giving it to someone who may have been included in the subject population in order to determine whether it is well written, clear, and inclusive of everything the researcher is looking for.

- **Reliability** is the repeatability of scientific observations. With reliability, the major question is: Can another researcher reproduce the study using a similar instrument and get similar results? A study may be reliable, but not valid. That is, the study may be able to be replicated and yet not answer the research question.

The type of data-collection technique used depends on the type of research the investigator wishes to conduct. If the researcher wants to establish a causal relationship, he or she should conduct one of the experimental studies. However, if the researcher is breaking new ground in a poorly understood area of practice, he or she may want to consider an exploratory study in a qualitative design.

Some examples of data-collection methods include:

- *Surveys:* The survey method gathers data from a relatively large number of cases at a particular time. Surveys can include interviews and questionnaire surveys. In either case, the questions should be well thought out to ensure that they answer the questions of the research study. The questions can be restricted, or closed ended, when the investigator only wants certain answers. For example, "Yes" and "No" answers fall into this category. It is a good idea to provide for unanticipated responses. Providing an "Other" category permits respondents to indicate what might be their most important response, one the questionnaire builder had not anticipated. Open-ended or **unrestricted questions** allow the participant to express a freer response in his or her own words. Open-ended questionnaires can be difficult to tabulate, and although they can be easier to write, it may be better to take additional time to write a closed-form type of questionnaire because it is easier to interpret and tabulate. When standardized questions are used in the interview process, this is referred to as a **structured interview.**

- *Observation:* Instead of asking questions, the investigator observes the participant.

  — In nonparticipant observation, the researcher is a neutral observer who does not interact with the participants.

  — In participant observation, the researcher may participate in the actions being observed but tries to maintain his or her objectivity.

  — Another type of observation is called **ethnography,** or **naturalistic observation.** Using this method of observation, the researcher observes, listens to, and sometimes converses with the subjects in as free and natural an atmosphere as possible. The assumption is that the most important behavior of individuals in groups is a dynamic process of complex interactions and consists of more than one set of facts, statistics, or even discrete incidents. A position of neutrality is important in this type of research.

- *Experimental study:* "This type of data collection technique provides a logical, systematic way to answer the question. If this is done under carefully controlled conditions, what will happen?" (Best and Kahn 1993, 162). There are many types of experimental studies, and a complete discussion would be too lengthy and complex for this introductory section. Experimentation is a sophisticated technique for the collection of data and may not be appropriate for the beginning investigator.

Selection of an Instrument

The **instrument,** also called a tool, is a consistent way to collect data. Many different types of instruments are used in research studies, and whatever type is used should be one that fits the purpose of the research.

Researchers sometimes use instruments that have been published in databases and occasionally publish their own instrument with their research. However, researchers should not develop an instrument until they have established that one does not already exist. If you decide to develop your own instrument, develop the questions carefully and be sure to test them to ensure that you are gathering what you need to answer the question in your research problem. It would be too costly and time-consuming to have to repeat a survey because a question or two had been neglected.

Selection of Samples

Another consideration in data collection is the selection of subjects for the study. For example, a study on health information departments in the United States could try to include every HIM department in the nation, but it would likely prove impractical and could be costly and time-consuming. The next best thing is to use a **sample.** When chosen correctly, samples are considered to be representative of the population.

Generally, there are two types of sampling techniques: probability sampling and non-probability sampling. Probability sampling uses some form of random selection. Probability sampling includes the following three types:

- Simple **random sampling:** This sampling technique involves choosing individuals from the population in such a way that every individual has an equal chance of being selected.

  Statistics books include a table of random numbers that can be used in the selection of random samples. In order to draw a random sample, the researcher should begin by assigning a number to each subject in the population. This number is dependent on the number of subjects in the population. For example, if there are 105 subjects in the population, the first subject would be numbered 001, the second 002, and so on with the final subject being number 105. Similarly, if there are 2,582 subjects in the population, the first subject would be numbered 0001, the second 0002, and the last subject 2,582. The researcher must begin by selecting subjects at random using the table of random numbers. This can be done by moving across or down the table, as long as the correct number of digits is selected. If the population contains 1,000 subjects, each time the researcher selects a subject, he must select four digits. If he comes across a number not included in the number of subjects (for example, the researcher comes across 8,569 but only has 1,000 subjects), this number is simply discarded and the he moves on to the next number.

  — In **systematic random sampling,** a systematic pattern is used with random sampling. For example, if you were choosing from a list of patients discharged during the past month, you might choose the first patient randomly and every fifth patient thereafter. In this sample, choice of the first patient determines the others.

- **Stratified random sampling:** To select a stratified random sample, divide the population into groups of similar individuals, called strata; choose a separate simple random sample (SRS) in each stratum; and then combine the SRSs to form the full sample. For example, you might want to make a selection based on gender, by patients with private insurance, or by separating hospitals by **bed size.**

- **Cluster sampling:** In this technique, the population is selected from groups, or clusters. For example, if the study includes HIM practitioners working in large cities, you first would choose the cities (the cluster) and then randomly choose the HIM practitioners from those cities. This is called two-stage cluster sampling.

Almost all qualitative research methods rely on nonprobability sampling. Nonprobability sampling does not involve a random sampling of the population. Nonprobability sampling includes:

- **Judgment sampling:** In judgment sampling, the researcher relies on his or her own judgment to select subjects for a study. For example, in a study on health information departments in acute care hospitals that are using an electronic health record, the researcher might use his or her judgment to select a specific hospital size for the study from among large, small, and medium-sized hospitals that use electronic health records.

- **Quota sampling:** In this type of sampling technique, the researcher first divides the population, as in stratified sampling, and then selects the number of subjects based on a specified proportion. In quota sampling, the selection of the sample is made by the researcher who has been given, or decides on, quotas to fill from the subgroup of the population. Continuing with the example of health information departments above, if 50 of the 100 hospitals in the state are using an electronic health record and 50 are not, the researcher may choose to base his or her study on 20 of the hospitals because that would be 20 percent of the total population of hospitals in the state.

- **Convenience sampling:** In this sampling technique, selection is based on the availability of subjects. Continuing with the example above, the researcher may decide to use only hospitals within a specific city or within a certain driving distance.

Introduction to Institutional Review Boards

Healthcare organizations that conduct research on human subjects are required to have an **Institutional Review Board** (IRB). The IRB is a committee whose primary responsibility is to protect the rights and welfare of research subjects. Professionals who serve on IRBs have extensive education and experience in clinical research. Most of these individuals have medical, doctoral, or other advanced degrees. IRB is a common term used in organizations; however, an institution may use whatever name it chooses. Some organizations refer to this group as an Independent Ethics Committee or Human Subjects Committee.

The IRB functions as a kind of ethics committee that focuses on what is right or wrong and what is undesirable in order to protect the rights and welfare of anyone participating in the research study. Because human subjects are involved, researchers are required to follow certain ethical principles that guide researcher behavior and morality. Research ethics provide:

- A structure for analysis and decision making

- Support and reminders for researchers to protect human subjects

- Workable definitions of benefits and risks

Risk versus benefit is critical in weighing the advantages of biomedical research. A benefit may be specific to the individual subject or to others as a result of the research.

Risks are concerned with the probability or extent of harm to the research subject. Probability of harm may be stated as 1 in 100 patients may experience a certain risk. Extent of harm may be a statement that indicates minor problems such as itchiness as a result of the treatment, or it may be a major effect of treatment such as liver failure that may result in death.

IRBs are responsible for reviewing the research procedures before the study is started and may require periodic reviews during the study. They may approve, revise, or deny requests for research in their facility. Any research on humans must be done carefully to ensure that subjects are not abused in any way. Referring to the earlier example of a study consisting of interviews with mothers of handicapped infants, although there would not be any physical pain to the mothers, questions asked in the study theoretically could cause the mothers emotional pain. The researcher must obtain permission from the IRB before any research study is started and prepare a plan for the research. This means that the researcher must have thought through the research very carefully, prepared any questionnaires, and decided how to select a sample and how to collect data in order to prepare the documentation necessary for the IRB, including informed consent forms for the subjects to read and sign.

In most cases, biomedical research requires that subjects must give an informed consent. Informed consent is a person's voluntary agreement to participate in research or to undergo a diagnostic, therapeutic, or preventive procedure. It is based on adequate knowledge and an understanding of relevant information provided by the investigators. In giving informed consent, subjects do not waive any of their legal rights nor do they release the investigator, sponsor, or institution from liability for negligence. Federal regulations require that certain information be provided each human subject, including:

- A statement that the study involves research, the purpose of the research, the expected time frame of subject participation, a description of the procedures to be followed, and the identification of procedures that are experimental

- A description of reasonably foreseeable risks or discomforts. The description must be accurate and reasonable, and subjects must be informed of previously reported adverse events.

- A description of the benefits to the subject or others who may reasonably benefit from the research

- A disclosure of any appropriate alternative procedures or courses of treatment that might be available. When appropriate, a statement that supportive care with no additional disease-specific treatment is an alternative.

- A statement describing the extent to which confidentiality of records identifying the subject will be maintained. The statement should include full disclosure and description of approved agencies, such as the FDA, that may have access to the records.

- For research involving more than minimal risk, an explanation as to whether any compensation or medical treatments are available if injury occurs, and, if so, what they consist of or where further information may be obtained

- An explanation of whom to contact for answers to pertinent questions about the research and whom to contact in the event of a research-related injury

- A statement that participation is voluntary, that refusal to participate will involve no penalty or loss of benefits, and that the subject may discontinue participation at any time

Federal regulations also require that informed consent be in a language that is understandable to the subject. The consent form must be translated into that language. Subjects who are not literate in their language must have an interpreter present to explain the study and to translate questions and answers between subject and investigator. A model consent form appears in figure 12.2.

Figure 12.2. Template for informed consent for research involving human subjects

Consent to Investigational Treatment or Procedure

I, _____ , hereby authorize or direct _____ or associates of his/her choosing to perform the following treatment or procedure (describe in general terms), upon _____ (myself).

The experimental (research) portion of the treatment or procedure is:

1. Purpose of the procedure or treatment

2. Possible appropriate alternative procedure or treatment (not to participate in the study is always an option)

3. Discomforts and risks reasonably to be expected

4. Possible benefits for subjects/society

5. Anticipated duration of subject's participation (including number of visits)

I hereby acknowledge that _____ has provided information about the procedure described above, about my rights as a subject, and he/she answered all questions to my satisfaction. I understand that I may contact him/her at phone number _____ should I have additional questions. He/she has explained the risks described above, and I understand them; he/she has also offered to explain all possible risks or complications.

I understand that, where appropriate, the US Food and Drug Administration may inspect records pertaining to this study. I understand further that records obtained during my participation in this study that may contain my name or other personal identifiers may be made available to the sponsor of this study. Beyond this, I understand that my participation will remain confidential.

I understand that I am free to withdraw my consent and participation in this project at any time after notifying the project director without prejudicing future care. No guarantee has been given to me concerning this treatment or procedure.

I understand that in signing this form, beyond giving consent, I am not waiving any legal rights that I might have and I am not releasing the investigator, the sponsor, or institution or its agents from any legal liability for damages that they might otherwise have.

In the event of injury resulting from participation in this study, I also understand that immediate medical treatment is available at _____ and that the costs of such treatment will be at my expense; financial compensation beyond that required by law is not available. Questions about this should be directed to the Office of Research Risks _____.

I have read and fully understand the consent form. I sign it freely and voluntarily. A copy has been given to me.

Source: AHIMA.

Privacy Considerations in Clinical and Biomedical Research

In response to a congressional mandate in the Health Insurance Portability and Account-ability Act (HIPAA), the Department of Health and Human Services issued regulations entitled Standards for Privacy of Individually Identifiable Health Information. Known as the Privacy Rule, it protects medical records and other **individually identifiable health information** from being used or disclosed in any form. Health information is individually identifiable if you can tell or could figure out to whom it refers by looking at it. The rule became effective on April 14, 2001, and organizations covered by the rule (covered enti-ties) were expected to be in compliance by April 14, 2003.

The Privacy Rule establishes a category of protected health information (PHI), which may be used or disclosed only in certain circumstances or under certain conditions. PHI is a subset of what is called individually identifiable health information. It includes what healthcare professionals typically regard as a patient's PHI, such as information in the patient's medial records as well as billing information for services rendered. PHI also includes identifiable health information about subjects of clinical research. Patient infor-mation considered "protected" is listed in figure 12.3.

The Privacy Rule defines the means by which human research subjects are informed of how their personal medical information will be used or disclosed. It also outlines their

Figure 12.3.   Examples of protected health information

The Privacy Rule allows covered entities to de-identify data by removing the following 18 elements that may be used to identify the individual or the individual's relatives, employers, or household members.

1. Names

2. All geographic subdivisions smaller than a state, including street address, city, county, precinct, and zip code, except for the initial three digits of a zip code if, according to the current publicly available data from the Bureau of the Census:

   a. The geographic unit formed by combining all zip codes with the same three initial digits contains more than 20,000 people

   b. The initial three digits of a zip code for all such geographic units containing 20,000 or fewer people are changed to 000

3. All elements of dates (except year) for dates directly related to an individual, including birth date, admission date, discharge date, date of death; and all ages over 89 and all elements of dates (including year) indicative of such age, except that such ages and elements may be aggregated into a single category of age 90 or older

4. Telephone numbers

5. Facsimile numbers

6. Electronic mail addresses

7. Social Security numbers

8. Medical record numbers

9. Health plan beneficiary numbers

10. Account numbers

11. Certificate/license numbers

12. Vehicle identifiers and serial numbers, including license plate numbers

13. Device identifiers and serial numbers

14. Web universal resource locators (URLs)

15. Internet protocol (IP) address numbers

16. Biometric identifiers, including fingerprints and voiceprints

17. Full-face photographic images and any comparable images

18. Any other unique identifying number, characteristic, or code, unless permitted by the Privacy Rule for re-identification

Source: AHIMA.

right to access the information. Further, it protects the privacy of individually identifiable information while ensuring that researchers continue to have access to the medical information they need to conduct their research. Investigators are permitted to use and disclose PHI for research with individual authorization or without individual authorization under limited circumstances.

A valid Privacy Rule authorization is an individual's signed permission allowing a covered entity to use or disclose the patient's PHI for the purpose(s) and to the recipient(s) stated in the authorization. When an authorization is obtained for biomedical research purposes, the Privacy Rule requires that it pertain only to a specific research study, not to future unspecified projects. The core elements of the Privacy Rule authorization are:

- A description of the PHI to be used or disclosed, identifying the information in a specific and meaningful manner

- The names or other specific identification of the person or persons authorized to make the requested use or disclosure

- The names or other specific identification of the person or persons to whom the covered entity may make the requested use or disclosure

- A description of each purpose of the requested use or disclosure

- An authorization expiration date or expiration event that relates to the individual or to the purpose of the use or disclosure

- The signature of the individual and the date. If the individual's legally authorized representative signs the authorization, a description of his or her authority to act for the individual also must be provided.

In addition, the authorization must include statements indicating:

- That the individual has the right to revoke the authorization at any time and must be provided with the procedure for doing so

- Whether treatment, payment, enrollment, or eligibility of benefits can be contingent upon authorization, including research-related treatment and consequences of refusing to sign the authorization, if applicable

- Any potential risk that the PHI will be redisclosed by the recipient and no longer protected by the Privacy Rule

Finally, the authorization must be written in plain language and a copy provided to the individual. A model HIPAA consent appears in figure 12.4; optional elements that may be included in the HIPAA consent are listed in figure 12.5.

Some facilities may also have a Research Protocol Monitoring Committee that reviews any research before and during the study to ensure that there are no adverse effects on the participants. It may even recommend closure of research that is not meeting safety standards, does not have scientific merit, or is not meeting the goals of the research.

Figure 12.4.   Model HIPAA consent: Required elements

**Authorization to Use or Disclose (Release) Health Information
That Identifies You for a Research Study**

If you sign this document, you give permission to ____(name of healthcare providers)____ at ____(name of covered entity)____ to use or disclose (release) your health information that identifies you for the research study described here:

(provide a description of the research study, such as title and purpose)

The health information that we may use or disclose (release) for this research includes:

The health information listed above may be used by and/or disclosed (released) to:

____(name of covered entity)____ is required by law to protect your health information. By signing this document, you authorize ____(name of covered entity)____ to use and/or disclose (release) your information for this research. Those persons who receive your health information may not be required by federal privacy laws (such as the Privacy Rule) to protect it and may share your information with others without your permission, if permitted by laws governing them.

Please note that (include the appropriate statement):

• You do not have to sign this authorization, but if you do not, you may not receive research-related treatment.

(when the research involves treatment and is conducted by the covered entity or when the covered entity provides healthcare solely for the purpose of creating protected health information to disclose to a researcher)

• (Name of covered entity) may not condition (withhold or refuse) treating you based upon whether you sign this authorization.

(when the research does not involve research-related treatment by the covered entity or when the covered entity is not providing healthcare solely for the purpose of creating protected health information to disclose to a researcher)

Please note that (include the appropriate statement):

• You may change your mind and revoke (take back) this authorization at any time, except to the extent that (name of covered entity) has already acted based on this authorization. To revoke this authorization, you must write to (name of covered entity and contact information).

(where the research study is conducted by an entity other than the covered entity)

• You may change your mind and revoke (take back) this authorization at any time. Even if you revoke this authorization, (name of persons at the covered entity involved in the research) may still use or disclose health information they already have obtained about you as necessary to maintain the integrity or reliability of the current research. To revoke this authorization, you must write to (name of covered entity and contact information).

This authorization does not have an expiration date.

Source: AHIMA.

Figure 12.5.   Model HIPAA consent: Optional elements

**Authorization to Use or Disclose (Release) Health Information
That Identifies You for a Research Study**

- Your health information will be used or disclosed when required by law.

- Your health information may be shared with a public health authority that is authorized by law to collect or receive such information for the purpose of preventing or controlling disease, injury, or disability, and conducting public health surveillance, investigations, or interventions.

- No publication or public presentation about the research described above will reveal your identity without another authorization from you.

- All information that does or can identify you is removed from your health information; the remaining information will no longer be subject to this authorization and may be used or disclosed for other purposes.

- **When the research for which the use or disclosure is made involves treatment and is conducted by a covered entity:** To maintain the integrity of this research study, you generally will not have access to your personal health information related to this research until the study is complete. At the conclusion of the research and at your request, you generally will have access to your health information that (name of covered entity) maintains in a designated record set that includes medical information or billing records used in whole or in part by your doctors or other healthcare providers at (name of covered entity) to make decisions about individuals. Access to your health information in a designated record set is described in the Notice of Privacy Practices provided to you by (name of covered entity). If it is necessary for your care, your health information will be provided to you or your physician.

- If you revoke this authorization, you may no longer be allowed to participate in the research described in this authorization.

Source: AHIMA.

Sample Size

Usually there is a trade-off between the desirability of a large sample and the feasibility of a small one. The ideal **sample size** is one that is large enough to serve as an adequate representation of the population about which the researcher wishes to generalize and small enough to be selected economically in terms of subject availability, expense in both time and money, and complexity of data analysis. Here are tips about sample size:

- The larger the sample, the smaller the magnitude of sampling error.

- Survey studies ordinarily have a larger sample size than experimental studies.

- Questionnaires that are mailed can have a response rate as low as 20 to 30 percent, so a large initial sample is recommended.

- When planning to have subgroups from the study population, begin with a large group to make sure you have enough participants for the subgroups.

- Subject availability and costs are legitimate considerations in determining appropriate sample size.

Analyzing the Data

In this step of the research process, the investigator tries to determine what the data disclose. Most researchers use a variety of techniques to describe the data. Two types of statistical applications are relevant to most studies:

- Descriptive statistics describe the data. Measures of central tendency and measures of variation are included in descriptive statistics. These are discussed in detail in chapter 10.

- Inferential statistics allow the researcher to make inferences about the population characteristics (parameters) from the sample's characteristics. Analysis of variance (ANOVA) and *t* tests are examples of inferential statistics that are discussed in chapter 13.

Statistics Software Packages

There are many software packages on the market to help researchers analyze their data. A search on the Internet will give you a listing of hundreds of free software packages. These packages can help the researcher produce descriptive statistics along with charts or graphs. One such package is Epi-Info, which is free software from the Centers for Disease Control and Prevention. It includes a program to create questionnaires along with allowing entry of data and analysis and creation of graphs and charts.

Another package, used in the pharmaceutical industry, is DecisionSite to help researchers predict a medication's chances for success. This software gives researchers the ability to combine lab data with patient demographics in order to help companies decide which drugs to develop and market.

SPSS (Statistical Package for Social Sciences) is a statistical package that supports many industries. It also is used by a variety of industries for its predictive analytics to help them make decisions.

Drawing Conclusions

Any conclusions reached from the study should be related to the hypothesis, or when using the qualitative approach, the identified problem. The results from each hypothesis should be described. Any limitations discovered during data analysis should be reported. For example, the study of health information departments mentioned earlier studied one city. That may be a limiting factor; that is, the conclusions may not apply to other geographical areas. In the presentation of the research findings, new hypotheses may be proposed if the data do not support the original hypothesis. Researchers usually include tables and graphs in this section of the research report to clarify and display the data.

Data Interpretation Issues

It has been said that statistics can tell us anything we want them to or that it is easy to lie with statistics. Unfortunately data can be misinterpreted in many ways. Sometimes misinterpretation is due to mistakes made in calculation or presentation of the data. Other times techniques are used so that data are purposely misconstrued. HIM professionals have an ethical obligation to report data honestly and accurately.

Misleading Presentation of Numbers

Statistics can be very powerful. Health information practitioners are generally the first individuals called upon to retrieve data for a facility; therefore, it is important for any "statistical communication" to be correct (Gelman, Nolan, 2002).

The easiest way to fabricate data is to simply make up the numbers. As reported by the United States Public Health Service, this is what happened in the case of Jon Sudbo. It was determined that he fabricated results in the reporting of information in a grant application and in its first-year progress report (Office of Research Integrity, October 9, 2007).

Another way to mislead people is to give misinformation, that is, to make a claim that is contradicted by the available statistics information. One must check the facts before asserting the information.

Ignoring the Baseline

Another common error that occurs is to compare raw numbers without adjusting the baseline. For example, if Hospital A and Hospital B each had 40 deaths last month, does this data provide the best indication of the level of care given at Hospital A and Hospital B? A better comparison would be to look at the number of total discharges and deaths during the last month well. If Hospital A had 200 total discharges and 40 deaths and Hospital B had 500 total discharges and 40 deaths, this additional data would change some inferences about each hospital. Knowing the case mix of each hospital (such as severity of cases and diagnoses) would provide additional data for a more accurate comparison.

Selection Bias

Statistical errors can also occur when a sample used in research does not represent the population. For example, if a report was generated on the length of stay of weekend admissions for the past year using as a sample patients admitted on Friday, Saturday, or Sunday and compared with a similar report from the previous year that used as a sample patients admitted on Saturday or Sunday, then the comparison would be biased. Comparison of the results in this example could be biased because the samples used did not represent the same days of the week.

Graphical Misrepresentations

Graphs can be manipulated to emphasize different points. For example, a bar graph can be designed so that the difference between bar heights is lessened. The smaller the increments on the y axis, the more definition there is between the different bars. A pie chart can be manipulated to pull one wedge away from the rest of the chart. This would bring greater emphasis to that portion of the pie chart even though there may not be significant differences from the rest of the chart. It is also important to be careful with three-dimensional graphs as these may misrepresent data, causing the data to appear smaller or larger.

Importance of Data Validation

Many statistical reports in healthcare settings are computer-generated. However, a computer can only calculate statistics from the data that are entered. When a statistical report is received, the HIM professional should examine it carefully. For example, he or she should verify the total number of discharges listed in a report from coded records and compare it against the total number of discharges according to the census data. Do the totals match? If not, it is important to find out why they do not. Many reports only report whole numbers.

The HIM professional may need to calculate certain statistics and carry them out to the second decimal place to make the information more valuable to administration or medical staff.

Ethical Guidelines in Statistics

The HIM professional has an obligation to follow ethical guidelines in statistical practice. Statistics play an important part in clinical and healthcare administrative decision making. Therefore statistical data collection, calculation, display, and interpretation must be appropriate and accurate. To help ensure data quality, HIM professionals should follow the edicts of the Institutional Review Board at their facilities and follow accepted ethical practice. When using statistics, HIM professionals must assure that they understand the capabilities and limitations of statistics. They must also use appropriate statistical methods and techniques for the question under study.

The American Statistical Association has developed Ethical Guidelines for Statistical Practice. They advocate for integrity in the professional work of researchers, particularly when private interests may inappropriately influence the reporting of statistics. Their guidelines in part read that statisticians should

- Present their findings and interpretations honestly and objectively
- Avoid untrue, deceptive, or undocumented statements
- Disclose any financial or other interests that may affect, or appear to affect, their professional statements

Hopefully, one's research will raise new questions about what should be studied and suggest needs for future research. The researcher should always include conclusions as to whether or not the problem is better understood or perhaps even resolved by the study.

Health information researchers provide other HIM professionals with knowledge and methods to answer questions and to decipher problems in the work setting. Researchers should be commended for their hard work because they must be very patient and unhurried. Research requires expertise and practice and is rarely spectacular work. However, it has contributed not only to a better place to practice health information management, but also to a better place to live and a greater understanding of the world around us.

Those students who would like to be involved in research and who need to develop skills in research should follow these steps:

1. Take at least one course in statistics and research methodologies.
2. Begin to read research studies in professional journals to see how others have performed their research.
3. Agree to work with a skilled health information researcher on a study to gain experience. You can find this information by contacting the author of a research study that you enjoyed reading. It is highly likely he or she will be performing another research study.
4. Learn how to present data effectively both in written form and verbally.

Statistics is the servant, not the master, of logic; it is a means rather than an end of research. "Unless basic assumptions are valid, unless the right data are carefully gathered, recorded, and tabulated, and unless the analysis and interpretations are logical, statistics can make no contribution to the search for truth" (Best and Kahn 1993, 316).

Exercise 12.1

Put the steps of the research process in order.

Order	Description
	Analyze the data
	Design the research
	Define the problem
	Draw conclusions
	Review the literature
	Collect the data

Exercise 12.2

Match the term with the definition.

1. _____ Ethnography
2. _____ Instrument
3. _____ Hypothesis
4. _____ Qualitative research
5. _____ Quantitative research
6. _____ Validity
7. _____ Quota sampling
8. _____ Reliability
9. _____ Judgment sampling
10. _____ Convenience sampling

A. Describes events, persons, and other information without the use of numerical data.

B. A method of observation where by the researcher observes, listens to, and sometimes converses with the subjects in a free and natural environment.

C. Uses numbers to describe a study, including comparisons and statistical data.

D. A technique that divides the population in question, then selects the number of subjects based on specified proportions.

E. A statement of the predicted outcome. The tentative answer to the question being asked.

F. The ability to repeat a scientific observation.

G. A tool, a consistent way to collect data.

H. The degree to which scientific observations actually measure or record what they claim to measure.

I. Selection is based on availability of subjects.

J. The researcher relies on his or her own decision to select subjects for study.

Chapter 12 Test

Complete the following exercises.

1. Which of the following is considered to be the search toward the solution of the problem?

   a. Fact
   b. Data
   c. Information
   d. Research

2. What are generally the two types of research?

   a. Basic and applied
   b. Scientific and hypothetical
   c. Theory and hypothesis
   d. Quantitative and qualitative

3. The type of research describing events, persons, and so on without the use of numerical data is called:

   a. Quantitative research
   b. Qualitative research
   c. Theoretical research
   d. Hypothetical research

4. The type of research that uses methods or numbers, including comparisons of the population and statistical analysis, to describe results is called:

   a. Quantitative research
   b. Qualitative research
   c. Theoretical research
   d. Hypothetical research

5. Which of the following refers to analysis that looks at the past?

   a. Theoretical analysis
   b. Hypothetical analysis
   c. Historical analysis
   d. Concurrent analysis

6. Which type of research tries to answer questions about what causes certain things to occur?

   a. Historical research
   b. Conclusive research
   c. Descriptive research
   d. Causal research

Chapter 12 Test (continued)

7. Which type of research provides data about the population you are studying and is also called statistical research?

   a. Historical research
   b. Conclusive research
   c. Descriptive research
   d. Causal research

8. Which type of research entails manipulation of a situation in some way in order to test a hypothesis?

   a. Correlational research
   b. Evaluation research
   c. Experimental research
   d. Hypothetical research

9. A statement of the predicted relationship of what the researcher is studying is called a(n):

   a. Educated guess
   b. Hypothesis
   c. Theory
   d. Essay

10. The degree to which scientific observations actually measure or record what they purport to measure is referred to as:

   a. Validity
   b. Reliability
   c. Integrity
   d. Theory

11. Which of the following is the repeatability of scientific observations?

   a. Validity
   b. Reliability
   c. Integrity
   d. Theory

12. Which data-collection method gathers data from a relatively large number of cases at a particular time?

   a. Observation
   b. Experimental study
   c. Survey
   d. Essay

(continued on next page)

Chapter 12 Test (continued)

13. This type of sample consists of individuals from the population chosen in such a way that every individual has an equal chance of being selected.

    a. Simple random sample
    b. Quota sample
    c. Cluster sample
    d. Judgment sample

14. In which type of sample does the researcher rely on his or her judgment to select the subjects?

    a. Simple random sample
    b. Quota sample
    c. Cluster sample
    d. Judgment sample

15. Statistics that describe the data are referred to as:

    a. Descriptive statistics
    b. Inferential statistics
    c. Measurement statistics
    d. Integral statistics

Chapter 13
Inferential Statistics in Healthcare

Key Terms

Analysis of variance (ANOVA)

Chi square

Confidence interval

Inferential statistics

Null hypothesis

Standard error of the mean

t test

Type I error

Type II error

Objectives

At the conclusion of this chapter, you should be able to:

- Define inferential statistics
- Interpret the standard error of the mean and confidence intervals
- Identify and describe the null hypothesis
- Understand the importance of t tests
- Interpret ANOVA
- Understand the significance of chi square

Inferential Statistics

Inferential statistics allow us to generalize from a sample to a population with a certain amount of confidence regarding our findings. Without inferential statistics, it would be very difficult, short of conducting a census, to describe the characteristics of a population. The ability to interpret inferential statistics requires a pre-existing understanding of descriptive statistical measures and computations.

Errors in sampling procedures are inevitable; even with random sampling, there is no guarantee that the sample drawn will be representative of the population. For this reason, inferential statistics are limited to certain amounts of confidence.

This chapter discusses the interpretation of common inferential statistical measures, including standard error of the mean, confidence intervals, the null hypothesis, *t* tests, ANOVA, and chi square.

It is not the intention of this chapter to replace your general statistics course requirement. This chapter merely provides a review of concepts you have learned in that course. An exhaustive explanation of these concepts, including mathematical computation, is beyond the scope of this book.

Standard Error of the Mean and Confidence Intervals

When trying to determine the characteristics of a population, the mean from one sample may not be sufficient because of random sampling error. A more accurate representation could be found by taking many large samples, calculating the mean for each sample, and then finding the standard deviation of all the sample means. This value is called the **standard error of the mean,** abbreviated SE_m, and comes from the standard deviation of many sample means. The graphical representation of all the sample means is a normal distribution when the sample size is reasonably large.

Finding the SE_m in the manner described above can be tedious, and it may not be realistic to find the SE_m of the sample means. For this reason statisticians have found a formula for approximating the SE_m from only one random sample ($SE_m = sd/sqrt(n)$). (A discussion of the theory leading to this formula is not covered in this book.) When the SE_m has been computed, it is generally reported in one of two ways.

1. The data may be displayed in research reports as follows:

$$\overline{X} = 150, sd = 10, n = 75, SE_m = 1.15$$

Where:

$$\overline{X} = \text{mean}$$

$$sd = \text{standard deviation}$$

$$n = \text{number of observations}$$

$$SE_m = \text{standard error of the mean}$$

Based on the characteristics of the normal curve and treating the SE_m as a margin of error, by adding the SE_m (1.15) to and subtracting it from the sample mean (150), it can be said that we are 68.3 percent sure that the interval

148.85 to 151.15 contains the population mean. This is called a **confidence interval** (abbreviated C.I.).

$$150 - 1.15 = 148.85$$
$$150 + 1.15 = 151.15$$

Similarly, it can be said that we are 95.5 percent sure that the interval 147.70 to 152.30 contains the population mean.

$$150 - (2 \times 1.15) = 147.70$$
$$150 + (2 \times 1.15) = 152.30$$

2. The data may be displayed in a research report as follows:

$$\overline{X} = 60, \; sd = 4, \; n = 16, \; SE_m = 1$$
$$68.3\% \; C.I. = 59 \; to \; 61$$
$$95.5\% \; C.I. = 58 \; to \; 62$$
$$99.7\% \; C.I. = 57 \; to \; 63$$

In this example, the confidence intervals have already been computed.

In a normal distribution, confidence intervals are computed by adding one standard error of the mean to and subtracting one from the mean, then adding two standard errors of the mean to and subtracting two from the mean, and so on. The percentages above come from a normal distribution:

68.3 percent of all scores in a normal distribution fall within + or – 1 standard deviation away from the mean

95.5 percent of all scores in a normal distribution fall within + or – 2 standard deviations away from the mean

99.7 percent of all scores in a normal distribution fall within + or – 3 standard deviations away from the mean

A confidence interval is the range of scores in which we are estimating the population mean to be. In the example above, the confidence intervals (C.I.) let us know, with a certain amount of confidence, where the mean will lie.

It is important to note that the larger the sample size, the more confidence there is in the mean and the smaller the chance for sampling errors, meaning a smaller SE_m. Further, the more homogenous a population (less variation), the smaller the SE_m. In fact, if a population were all the same (no variation) the SE_m would be zero.

The Null Hypothesis

The **null hypothesis** states that the difference between two population means is zero. This statement is generally made based on two sample means. For example, let's suppose we obtain a sample of the heights of 15-year-old girls at high school A and a second sample of the heights of 15-year-old girls at school B. These are the means:

High school A: $\overline{x} = 5.7$ ft.

High school B: $\overline{x} = 5.6$ ft.

From these results, it would appear that 15-year-old girls at high school A are taller than 15-year-old girls at high school B. However, this may not be true; in fact, the difference may be due to errors in sampling and the mean of the heights of girls at high school A (population mean) may equal the heights of girls at high school B (population mean). This is a statement of a null hypothesis.

The null hypothesis can be expressed as follows:

$H_0: \mu_1 - \mu_2 = 0$

H_0 represents the null hypothesis.

μ_1 represents the population mean for group 1.

μ_2 represents the population mean for group 2.

When conducting research, most researchers are searching for differences in population means and are therefore not looking to confirm the null hypothesis. In fact, most research is carried out to reject the null hypothesis. Therefore, researchers may develop an alternative hypothesis to test against the null. The alternative hypothesis can be expressed in one of three ways:

$H_1 = \mu_1 > \mu_2$

H_1 represents the alternative hypothesis.

μ_1 represents the population mean for group 1, hypothesized to be larger than group 2.

μ_2 represents the population mean for group 2, hypothesized to be smaller than group 1.

or

$H_1 = \mu_1 < \mu_2$

H_1 represents the alternative hypothesis.

μ_1 represents the population mean for group 1, hypothesized to be smaller than group 2.

μ_2 represents the population mean for group 2, hypothesized to be larger than group 1.

or

$H_1 = \mu_1 \neq \mu_2$

H_1 represents the alternative hypothesis.

μ_1 represents the population mean for group 1, hypothesized to be different from group 2 without sufficient information to determine which group is larger.

μ_2 represents the population mean for group 2, hypothesized to be different from group 1 without sufficient information to determine which group is larger.

The first alternative hypothesis states that group 1 is larger than group 2; this would be the same as the samples would imply, that 15-year-old girls from high school A are taller than 15-year-old girls from high school B. The second alternative hypothesis states that group 1 is smaller than group 2; this would indicate the samples do not represent the population, and that 15-year-old girls from high school A are not taller than 15-year-old girls from high school B. The third alternative hypothesis states that group 1 and group 2 are different, but there is not enough information to determine which population of girls has the higher mean height.

Because there is always a chance that the null hypothesis is true, testing it will lead to a probability (p) that it is true. The smaller the p value (probability that the null hypothesis is true), the more evidence that we should reject the null hypothesis. As a rule of thumb accepted by most statisticians in hypothesis testing, if the probability that the null hypothesis is true is 5 percent or less, the null hypothesis is rejected.

In hypothesis testing, rejecting the null hypothesis with this level of confidence is, in effect, describing the relationship between the means as statistically significant. This is generally the manner in which the null hypothesis is discussed in academic journals.

Probabilities of the null hypothesis are expressed as follows:

$p < 5\%$ The probability that the null hypothesis is true is less than 5 percent.

$p < 1\%$ The probability that the null hypothesis is true is less than 1 percent.

$p < 0.1\%$ The probability that the null hypothesis is true is less than 0.1 percent.

Where: p = the probability that the null hypothesis is true given the values present in the sample. Remember, we are generalizing from a sample to make conclusions about the population.

These different probabilities represent different statistical significance levels; the lower the percentage that the null hypothesis is true, the more significant the finding. Thus, a $p \leq 0.1\%$ is more significant a finding than a $p \leq 5\%$.

Dealing with levels of uncertainty in hypothesis testing creates two types of errors: Type I errors and Type II errors. A **Type I error** occurs when the null hypothesis is rejected, yet it is actually true. A **Type II error** occurs when the null hypothesis is not rejected, yet it is false. Following are examples of both types of errors.

Type I Error

According to the National Cancer Institute, a woman's chance of being diagnosed with breast cancer from age 50 through age 59 is 2.38 percent. With this knowledge, going to see a doctor because of a lump on her breast presents a risk that the doctor will diagnose the patient with breast cancer even if she does not have breast cancer. Consider the following null hypothesis: there is no difference between women diagnosed with breast cancer and women not diagnosed with breast cancer. Rejecting the null hypothesis in this instance would be assuming that the doctor will not diagnose her with breast cancer as there is a difference between the two populations (women diagnosed with breast cancer and women not diagnosed with breast cancer). However, if she is diagnosed with breast cancer, this would be an example of a Type I error. Simply said, the patient could receive a positive test result when, in fact, she does not have breast cancer.

Type II Error

A Type I error is controlled by the researcher setting the acceptable error rate. A Type II error is driven by the sample size and the particular test used. Suppose a drug company has developed a new drug for a serious disease. Suppose that, in reality, the new drug is effective. If, however, the null hypothesis is not rejected because the drug company selected a level of significance that is too high, the results of the study will have to be described as insignificant and the drug may not receive government approval (Pyrczak, 2003, 83). This is an example of a Type II error.

When describing the null hypothesis, it is never "accepted." Rather, we say "reject the null hypothesis" or "fail to reject the null hypothesis."

The *t* Test

A *t* **test** is an example of a test of the null hypothesis to determine if a set of results is statistically significant. As mentioned previously, for the results to be considered statistically significant, the probability that the null hypothesis is true should be 5 percent or less. The results of a *t* test can be written several ways. Consider the following example.

Example:

Group	$\bar{x}$	Standard Deviation (sd)	n
A	5.3	1.6	10
B	6.6	1.0	10

With this group of data, the results of the *t* test (computed using computer software or a calculator) can be written as follows:

The null hypothesis: There is no difference between the groups.

H_0: $\mu_1 - \mu_2 = 0$ (the difference between the means is zero)

1. Statistically significant ($t = 2.18$, $df = 18$, $p < 0.05$)

2. Statistically significant at the 0.05 level ($t = 2.18$, $df = 18$)

3. Reject H_0 at the 0.05 level ($t = 2.18$, $df = 18$)

Where: t = the value produced by the *t* test

df = The degrees of freedom are found by taking $n - 1$ for the number of groups. In the sample above, there are two groups, therefore:

$df = (n_1 - 1) + (n_2 - 1)$

$df = (10 - 1) + (10 - 1) = 18$

$df = 18$

Statements 1 through 3 above all reject the null hypothesis and say that there is a statistically significant difference between the population means of Group A and Group B ($5.3 - 6.6 = -1.3$).

However, the sample data may not support the conclusion that there is a statistically significant difference between the means. Consider the following example.

Example:

Group	$\bar{x}$	Standard Deviation (sd)	n
A	25	3	8
B	24	3	8

H_0: $\mu_1 - \mu_2 = 0$ (the difference between the means is zero)

1. Not statistically significant ($t = 0.67$, $df = 14$, $p > 0.05$)

2. H_0 is not rejected at the 0.05 level ($t = 0.67$, $df = 14$)

These statements do not reject the null hypothesis and say that the difference between the sample means is not statistically significant (25 − 24 = 1). The null hypothesis is not rejected because the probability of the null hypothesis actually occurring is greater than 5 percent; for this reason, the difference between the means is not statistically significant.

Example:

Group	$\bar{x}$	Standard Deviation (sd)	n
A	18	2.5	7
B	17	8	7

The null hypothesis: There is no difference between the groups.

H_0: $\mu_1 - \mu_2 = 0$ (the difference between the means is zero)

($t = 0.32$, $df = 12$, $p > 0.05$) Do not reject the null hypothesis.

Exercise 13.1

Given the information in the example above, would you reject the null hypothesis or not? How would you state your findings?

It is important to note that understanding the computation involved in testing the null hypothesis is reserved for an advanced statistics course and is not part of the daily activities of a healthcare practitioner. How to interpret the results of these tests, however, is important. For this reason, the next two sections on ANOVA and chi square are briefly introduced.

ANOVA

Although *t* tests are used to test the difference between two means, an **analysis of variance** (ANOVA) test is used to test the differences among more than two means. Sometimes ANOVA is referred to as an *F* test. In the special case when only two means are tested, the *F* test will yield a *p*-value that is the same as a *t* test for testing the difference between two population means.

In the following example, the means from four samples are listed. Using ANOVA will test to determine if any of six differences among the means is statistically significant.

	LOS Group 1: Patients with Private Insurance	LOS Group 2: Patients with Medicare/Medicaid
Males	$\bar{x} = 10$	$\bar{x} = 23$
Females	$\bar{x} = 15$	$\bar{x} = 17$

Males with Private Insurance (Group A): $\bar{x} = 11$

Males with Medicare/Medicaid (Group B): $\bar{x} = 19$

Females with Private Insurance (Group C): $\bar{x} = 17$

Females with Medicare/Medicaid (Group D): $\bar{x} = 20$

Differences tested by ANOVA:

1. Between A and B
2. Between A and C
3. Between A and D
4. Between B and C
5. Between B and D
6. Between C and D

This is the power of ANOVA, the ability to test many differences among means at once. If the results from an ANOVA are statistically significant (reject the null hypothesis that at least one of the pairs of means is different), the researcher's next step is to figure out what differences are significant. However, if the results are not statistically significant (the null hypothesis is not rejected), the work is done.

Chi Square

Chi square (represented by the symbol χ^2) is a test of significance that deals with nominal data and frequencies, specifically data where the standard deviation and mean are not meaningful descriptions. Note that calculation is possible, just not meaningful. Using computer software to conduct a chi square test is simple and quickly yields results. Consider the following example.

Example: Employees at a large healthcare facility were randomly asked whether they smoked and whether they had parents who smoked. The results of the 150 employees sampled were:

	Parents Who Smoke	**Parents Who Do Not Smoke**
Employee smokes	45	25
Employee does not smoke	30	50

These data in this table suggest that those employees with parents who did not smoke were likelier not to smoke (50 vs. 25) than were those employees with parents who smoked (30 vs. 45). From this sample alone, there appears to be a relationship between smoking and having parents who smoke. However, there is a possibility that the null hypothesis, that the relationship does not exist in this population, is true. A chi square test can determine whether the relationship is statistically significant. A chi square test using the values above yielded these results:

$$\chi^2 = 10.71, df = 1, p < 0.01$$

Based on the results, there is a less than 1 percent chance that the null hypothesis is true. Said another way, the results are statistically significant; there is a relationship between employees who do not smoke having parents who do not smoke.

Notice below that the degrees of freedom are determined differently for chi square. The degrees of freedom are found by taking $(r-1) \times (c-1)$ for the number of categories where r = the number of rows and c = the number of columns.

$$df = (r-1)$$
$$df = (2-1) = 1$$
$$df = 1$$

Exercise 13.2

In the following two questions, identify which choices would be considered descriptive statistics and which would be considered inferential statistics.

1. Of 500 randomly selected people in New York City, 210 people had O+ blood.
   a. "42 percent of the people in New York City have O+ blood." Is the statement descriptive statistics or inferential statistics?
   b. "58 percent of the people of New York City do not have type O+ blood." Is the statement descriptive statistics or inferential statistics?
   c. "42 percent of all people living in New York State have type O+ blood." Is the statement descriptive statistics or inferential statistics?

2. On the last three Friday evenings, City Hospital diagnosed a number of heroin overdoses. There were four on January 14, 20XX, two on January 21, 20XX, and six on January 28, 20XX.
   a. "City Hospital averaged four heroin overdoses in their ER for the last three Friday evenings."
   b. "City Hospital never has more than six heroin overdoes on Friday evenings."
   c. "Friday nights are the busiest time for heroin overdoses at City Hospital."

Chapter 13 Test

1. Define inferential statistics.

2. Explain the difference between descriptive and inferential statistics.

3. Create a null hypothesis for the following research questions:
   a. What are the differences between emergency room shifts on medication errors?
   b. On a clinical trial of a new drug, what will be the effects over a currently used drug?

4. How could you reword these research hypotheses to null hypotheses?
   a. Smoking during pregnancy increases the risk of a child being born prematurely.
   b. Regular exercise in older adults decreases blood pressure levels.

5. Based on the results below, how would you describe the relationship between heart attack patients being treated with aspirin and whether or not they lived?

	Male Heart Attack Patients Treated with Aspirin	Male Heart Attack Patients Not Treated with Aspirin
Males who lived	15	4
Males who did not live	2	8

$$\chi^2 = 8.34, df = 1, p \leq 0.01$$

(continued on next page)

Chapter 13 Test (continued)

6. Using the following information, determine if the differences between the means are significant.

   Medical Terminology Class

   Group A = Number of word elements remembered by students using flash cards

   Group B = Number of word elements remembered by students not using flash cards

Group	$\bar{x}$	Standard Deviation (sd)	n
A	75	2.0	10
B	50	3.5	10

   The null hypothesis: There is no difference between the groups.

   H_0: $\mu_1 - \mu_2 = 0$ (the difference between the means is zero)

   $(t = 2.50, df = 18, p < 0.05)$

7. Given the following p values, which would be considered more significant?

   a. $p \leq 0.3$
   b. $p \leq 0.02$
   c. $p \leq 0.25$

8. Given the following null hypothesis, give an example of a Type I error.

   H_0: There is no difference between the number of males or females who go to their primary care physician for an annual exam.

9. Given the following null hypothesis, give an example of a Type II error.

   H_0: There is no difference in the level of understanding of this chapter between students who have previously taken a statistics course and students who have not previously taken a statistics course.

10. Given the following information, determine the 68.3 percent, 95.5 percent, and 99.7 percent confidence intervals.

    $\bar{x} = 4.33, SE_m = 3$

References

AHIMA e-HIM Work Group. 2003. Practice brief: Electronic document management as a component of the electronic health record. http://library.ahima.org/xpedio/groups/public/documents/ahima/bok1_021594.hcsp?dDocName=bok1_021594.

AHIMA e-HIM Work Group. 2003. Practice brief: E-mail as a provider–Patient electronic communication medium and its impact on the electronic health record. http://library.ahima.org/xpedio/groups/public/documents/ahima/bok1_021588.hcsp.

AHIMA e-HIM Work Group on Health Information in a Hybrid Environment. 2003. Practice brief: The complete medical record in a hybrid environment. http://library.ahima.org/xpedio/groups/public/documents/ahima/bok1_022142.hcsp.

AHIMA e-HIM Work Group on Implementing Electronic Signatures. 2003. Practice brief: Implementing electronic signatures. http://library.ahima.org/xpedio/groups/public/documents/ahima/bok1_045551.hcsp?dDocName=bok1_045551.

American Statistical Association. 1999. Ethical Guidelines For Statistical Practice. http://www.amstat.org/about/ethicalguidelines.cfm.

Ball, C.N., and J. Conner-Linton. 2003. WebChi Square Calculator. http://www.georgetown.edu/faculty/ballc/webtools/web_chi.html. (site discontinued)

Best, J., and J. Kahn. 1993. *Research in Education.* 7th ed. Boston: Allyn and Bacon.

Centers for Disease Control and Prevention. 2005. Nosocomial Infections Surveillance System (NNIS). http://www.cdc.gov/nhsn.

Centers for Disease Control and Prevention. 2007. Leading Causes of Deaths. http://www.cdc.gov/nchs/fastats/lcod.htm.

Centers for Disease Control and Prevention. 2010. National Healthcare Safety Network. http://www.cdc.gov/nhsn/.

Department of Health and Human Services. 2004. Clinical Research and the HIPAA Privacy Rule. NIH Publication Number 04-5495. Washington, DC: HHS. Available online from http://privacyruleandresearch.nih.gov/pdf/clin_research.pdf.

Department of Health and Human Services. 2004. HIPAA Authorization for Research. NIH Publication Number 04-5529. Washington, DC: HHS. Available online from http://privacyruleandresearch.nih.gov/pdf/authorization.pdf.

Department of Health and Human Services. 2004. Protecting Personal Health Information in Research: Understanding the HIPAA Privacy Rule. NIH Publication Number 03-5388. Washington, DC: HHS. Available online from http://privacyruleandresearch.nih.gov/pdf/HIPAA_Booklet_4-14-2003.pdf.

Dinman, S. 1996. A guide to nursing research. *Plastic Surgical Nursing* 16(2).

Dunn, R. 1999. *Finance Principles for the Health Information Manager.* Chicago: AHIMA.

Dunn, R. 2002. Turning production data into management tools. *Journal of AHIMA* 73(9):60–66.

Dunn, R. 2003. Calculating costs for accounting of disclosures. *Journal of AHIMA* 74(5):65–66.

Freund, John E., and Gary A. Simon. 1995. *Statistics: A First Course,* 6th ed. New Jersey: Prentice-Hall.

Garner, J. 1985. Guideline for Prevention of Surgical Wound Infections. Hospital Infections Program. Centers for Infectious Diseases Center for Disease Control. http://wonder.cdc.gov/wonder/prevguid/p0000420/p0000420.asp#head004003000000000.

Gauvreau, K., and M. Pagano. 1993. *Principles of Biostatistics.* Belmont, CA: Duxbury Press.

Gelman, A., and D. Nolan. 2002. *Teaching Statistics: A Bag of Tricks.* New York: Oxford University Press. Also available online at http://stat.columbia.edu/~gelman/bag-of-tricks/chap10.pdf.

Jacobsen, Kathryn H. 2012. *Introduction to Health Research Methods: A Practical Guide.* Sudbury, MA: Jones and Bartlett.

Johns, M., ed. 2011. *Health Information Management Technology: An Applied Approach,* 3rd ed. Chicago: AHIMA.

Johnson, T., and H. Neill. 2001. *Mathematics.* Chicago: Contemporary Books.

Koch, Doreen. 2011. Interview April 21. Promise Regional Medical Center, Hutchinson, KS.

Lane, D.M. 2005. *HyperStat Online Statistics Textbook.* http://davidmlane.com/hyperstat/.

LaTour, K., and S. Eichenwald Maki. 2009. *Health Information Management: Concepts, Principles, and Practice,* 3rd ed. Chicago: AHIMA.

Lorence, D. 1999. Productivity: How do you measure up? *Journal of AHIMA* 70(5):35–39.

Malone, S. 1997. Staffing to volume in integrated delivery networks. *Journal of AHIMA* 68(9):42–48.

Miller, P.J., and F.L. Waterstraat. 2004. Apples to apples: Using autobenchmarking to measure productivity. *Journal of AHIMA* 75(1):44–49.

Moore, D.S. 2004. *The Basic Practice of Statistics,* 3rd ed. New York: W.H. Freeman and Company.

National Cancer Institute. 2010. Probability of Breast Cancer in American Women. http://www.cancer.gov/cancertopics/factsheet/detection/Fs5_6.pdf.

National Center for Health Statistics. 2003. National Vital Statistics System. http://www.cdc.gov/nchs/nvss.htm.

National Center for Health Statistics. 2007. Deaths and Mortality (US) Final Data for 2007. http://www.cdc.gov/nchs/fastats/deaths.htm.

National Center for Health Statistics. 2009. National Vital Statistics Reports. Deaths: Final Data for 2006. http://www.cdc.gov/nchs/data/nvsr/nvsr57/nvsr57_14.pdf.

National Conference of State Legislatures, 2009. Certificate of Need: State Health Laws and Programs. http://www.ncsl.org/default.aspx?tabid=14373.

National Institutes of Health, Public Health Service. 1994. *Statistics and Epidemiology for Cancer Registries.* SEER Program Self-Instructional Manual for Cancer Registrars, Book 7. Publication No. 94-3766. Washington, DC: US Department of Health and Human Services.

National Program of Cancer Registries. United States Cancer Statistics. 1999–2007 Cancer Incidence and Mortality Data. http://apps.nccd.cdc.gov/uscs/.

Office of Research Integrity. 2007. Findings of scientific misconduct. Case Summary—Jon Sudbo. *Federal Register* 72(194). Available online from http://ori.dhhs.gov/misconduct/cases/Sudbo.shtml.

Osborn, C. 2000. *Statistical Applications for Health Information Management.* Gaithersburg, MD: Aspen.

Pronovost, P., D. Angus, T. Dorman, K. Robinson, T. Dremsizov, and T. Young. 2002. Physician staffing patterns and clinical outcomes in critically ill patients. *JAMA* 288(17): 2151–2162.

Pyrczak, F. 2003. *Making Sense of Statistics: A Conceptual Overview.* Los Angeles: Pyrczak Publishing.

Reswick, J. 1994. What constitutes valid research? Qualitative vs. quantitative research. *Journal of Rehabilitation Research and Development* 31(2).

Rudner, L., and W.D. Schafer. 1999. How to write a scholarly research report. *Practical Assessment, Research & Evaluation* 6(13). http://pareonline.net/getvn.asp?v=6&n=13.

Salkind, N. 2004. *Statistics for People Who (Think They) Hate Statistics.* Thousand Oaks, CA: Sage Publications.

Seltzer, William. 2005. Official Statistics and Statistical Ethics: Selected Issues. Paper presented at the International Statistical Institute, 55th Session, Sydney, Australia. Available online from http://unstats.un.org/unsd/methods/statorg/links.asp.

Tobacco Outlook Report, Economic Research Service, US Department of Agriculture. Available at http://www.infoplease.com/ipa/A0908700.html.

US Census Bureau. National and State Population Estimates 2000–2007. http://www.census.gov/popest/states/NST-ann-est2007.html.

US Department of Health and Human Services. Hospital Compare. http://www.hospitalcompare.hhs.gov/Hospital/Search/Welcome.asp?version=default&browser=IE%7C6%7CWinXP&language=English&defaultstatus=0&pagelist=Home.

WebMD. 2010. Types of Anesthesia. http://www.webmd.com/pain-management/tc/anesthesia-types-of-anesthesia.

Youngs, Kelene. 2011. Interview April 22. Promise Regional Medical Center, Hutchinson, KS.

Appendix A
Formulas

Formulas Listed Alphabetically by Name

Adjusted Hospital Autopsy Rate (p. 101) [Chapter 7]

$$\frac{Total\ hospital\ autopsies \times 100}{Total\ number\ of\ deaths\ of\ hospital\ patients\ whose\ bodies\ are\ available\ for\ autopsy}$$

Anesthesia Death Rate (p. 80) [Chapter 6]

$$\frac{Total\ deaths\ caused\ by\ anesthetic\ agents \times 100}{Total\ number\ of\ anesthetics\ administered}$$

Average (p. 20) [Chapter 2]

$$\frac{Sum\ of\ all\ the\ values}{Number\ of\ all\ the\ values\ involved} = \overline{X}$$

Average Daily Inpatient Census (p. 38) [Chapter 3]

$$\frac{Total\ inpatient\ service\ days\ for\ a\ period\ (excluding\ newborns)}{Total\ number\ of\ days\ in\ the\ period}$$

Average Daily Inpatient Census for a Patient Care Unit (p. 39) [Chapter 3]

$$\frac{Total\ inpatient\ service\ days\ for\ the\ unit\ for\ the\ period}{Total\ number\ of\ days\ in\ the\ period}$$

Average Daily Newborn Census (p. 39) [Chapter 3]

$$\frac{Total\ newborn\ inpatient\ service\ days\ for\ a\ period}{Total\ number\ of\ days\ in\ the\ period}$$

Average Length of Stay (p. 63) [Chapter 5]

$$\frac{Total\ length\ of\ stay\ (discharge\ days)}{Total\ discharges\ (including\ deaths)}$$

Average Newborn Length of Stay (p. 64) [Chapter 5]

$$\frac{Total\ newborn\ discharge\ days}{Total\ newborn\ discharges\ (including\ deaths)}$$

Bed Occupancy Ratio (p. 46) [Chapter 4]

$$\frac{Total\ inpatient\ service\ days\ in\ a\ period \times 100}{Total\ bed\ count\ days\ in\ the\ period\ (Bed\ count \times Number\ of\ days\ in\ the\ period)}$$

Bed Turnover Rate, Direct Formula (p. 53) [Chapter 4]

$$\frac{Number\ of\ discharges\ (including\ deaths)\ for\ a\ period}{Average\ bed\ count\ during\ the\ period}$$

Bed Turnover Rate, Indirect Formula (p. 53) [Chapter 4]

$$\frac{Occupancy\ rate \times Number\ of\ days\ in\ a\ period}{Average\ length\ of\ stay}$$

Cancer Mortality Rate (p. 90) [Chapter 6]

$$\frac{Number\ of\ cancer\ deaths\ during\ a\ period \times 100,000}{Total\ number\ in\ population\ at\ risk}$$

Case Fatality Rate (p. 73) [Chapter 6]

$$\frac{Number\ of\ people\ who\ die\ of\ a\ disease\ in\ a\ specified\ period \times 100}{Number\ of\ people\ who\ have\ the\ disease}$$

Case-mix (p. 158) [Chapter 9]

$$\frac{Sum\ of\ the\ weights\ of\ MS\text{-}DRGs\ (Medicare\ severity\ diagnosis\text{-}related\ groups)\ for\ patients\ discharged\ during\ a\ given\ period}{Total\ number\ of\ patients\ discharged}$$

Cesarean-section Rate (p. 124) [Chapter 8]

$$\frac{Total\ number\ of\ C\text{-}sections\ performed\ in\ a\ period \times 100}{Total\ number\ of\ deliveries\ in\ the\ period\ (including\ C\text{-}sections)}$$

Complication Rate (p. 123) [Chapter 8]

$$\frac{Total\ number\ of\ complications\ for\ a\ period \times\ 100}{Total\ number\ of\ discharges\ in\ the\ period}$$

Consultation Rate (p. 127) [Chapter 8]

$$\frac{Total\ number\ of\ patients\ receiving\ a\ consultation \times 100}{Total\ number\ of\ patients\ discharged}$$

Fetal Autopsy Rate (p. 105) [Chapter 7]

$$\frac{Autopsies\ performed\ on\ intermediate\ and\ late\ fetal\ deaths\ for\ a\ period \times 100}{Total\ intermediate\ and\ late\ fetal\ deaths\ for\ the\ same\ period}$$

Fetal Death Rate (p. 88) [Chapter 6]

$$\frac{Total\ number\ of\ intermediate\ and/or\ late\ fetal\ deaths\ for\ a\ period \times 100}{Total\ number\ of\ live\ births\ +\ Intermediate\ and\ late\ fetal\ deaths\ for\ the\ period}$$

Gross Autopsy Rate (p. 96) [Chapter 7]

$$\frac{Total\ autopsies\ on\ inpatient\ deaths\ for\ a\ period \times 100}{Total\ inpatient\ deaths\ for\ the\ period}$$

Gross (Hospital) Death Rate (p. 73) [Chapter 6]

$$\frac{Number\ of\ inpatient\ deaths\ (including\ NB)\ in\ a\ period\ \times 100}{Number\ of\ discharges\ (including\ A\&C\ and\ NB\ deaths)\ in\ the\ same\ period}$$

Infection Rate (p. 117) [Chapter 8]

$$\frac{Total\ number\ of\ infections \times 100}{Total\ number\ of\ discharges\ (including\ deaths)\ for\ the\ period}$$

Labor Productivity (p. 148) [Chapter 9]

$$Completed\ work = Total\ work\ output - Defective\ work$$

$$Labor\ productivity = \frac{Completed\ work}{Hours\ worked\ to\ produce\ total\ work\ output}$$

Maternal Death Rate (p. 82) [Chapter 6]

$$\frac{\textit{Number of direct maternal deaths for a period} \times 100}{\textit{Number of obstetrical discharges (including deaths) for the period}}$$

Mean (p. 176) [Chapter 10]

$$\frac{\textit{Total sum of all the values}}{\textit{Number of values involved}} = \overline{X}$$

or

$$\frac{\Sigma\ scores}{N} = \frac{\textit{Sum of all scores}}{\textit{Total number of scores}}$$

Net Autopsy Rate (p. 98) [Chapter 7]

$$\frac{\textit{Total autopsies on inpatient deaths for a period} \times 100}{\textit{Total inpatient deaths} - \textit{Unautopsied coroners' or medical examiners' cases}}$$

Net Death Rate (p. 76) [Chapter 6]

$$\frac{\textit{Total number of inpatient deaths (including NB) minus deaths} < 48\ \textit{hours for a given period} \times 100}{\textit{Total number of discharges (including NB deaths) minus deaths} < 48\ \textit{hours from the same period}}$$

Newborn Autopsy Rate (p. 104) [Chapter 7]

$$\frac{\textit{Newborn autopsies for a period} \times 100}{\textit{Total newborn deaths for the period}}$$

Newborn Bassinet Occupancy Ratio (p. 51) [Chapter 4]

$$\frac{\textit{Total newborn inpatient service days for a period} \times 100}{\textit{Total newborn bassinet count} \times \textit{Number of days in the period}}$$

Newborn Mortality Rate (p. 86) [Chapter 6]

$$\frac{\textit{Total number of newborn deaths for a period} \times 100}{\textit{Total number of newborn discharges (including deaths) for the period}}$$

Nosocomial Infection Rate (p. 117) [Chapter 8]

$$\frac{\textit{Total number of nosocomial infections for a period} \times 100}{\textit{Total number of discharges, including deaths, for the same period}}$$

Other Rates (p. 129) [Chapter 8]

$$\frac{Number\ of\ times\ something\ happened \times 100}{Number\ of\ times\ something\ could\ have\ happened}$$

Payback Period (p. 154) [Chapter 9]

$$\frac{Total\ cost\ of\ project}{Annual\ incremental\ cash\ flow}$$

Postoperative Death Rate (p. 77) [Chapter 6]

$$\frac{Total\ number\ of\ deaths\ (within\ 10\ days\ after\ surgery) \times 100}{Total\ number\ of\ patients\ who\ were\ operated\ on\ for\ the\ period}$$

Postoperative Infection Rate (p. 120) [Chapter 8]

$$\frac{Total\ number\ of\ infections\ in\ clean\ surgical\ cases\ for\ a\ period \times 100}{Number\ of\ surgical\ operations\ for\ the\ period}$$

Rate (p. 19) [Chapter 2]

$$Rate = \frac{Part}{Base}, \text{ or } R = \frac{P}{B}$$

Return on Investment (p. 154) [Chapter 9]

$$\frac{Average\ annual\ incremental\ cash\ flow}{Total\ cost\ of\ the\ project}$$

Staffing Level (p. 148) [Chapter 9]

$$\frac{Patient\ encounters}{Productivity} = Number\ of\ FTEs\ needed$$

Standard Deviation (p. 185) [Chapter 10]

$$SD = \sqrt{\frac{\sum(X - \overline{X})^2}{(N-1)}}$$

Unit Labor Costs (p. 138) [Chapter 9]

$$\frac{Total\ (sum)\ employee\ compensation}{Total\ (sum)\ employee\ annual\ productivity}$$

Variance (p. 182) [Chapter 10]

$$s^2 = \frac{(X_1 - \overline{X})^2 + (X_2 - \overline{X})^2 + (X_3 - \overline{X})^2 \ and\ so\ on}{N-1}$$

Vital Statistics Infant Mortality Rate (p. 86) [Chapter 6]

$$\frac{Number\ of\ infant\ deaths\ (neonatal\ and\ postneonatal)\ during\ a\ period \times 1,000}{Number\ of\ live\ births\ during\ the\ period}$$

Vital Statistics Maternal Mortality Rate (p. 82) [Chapter 6]

$$\frac{Number\ of\ deaths\ attributed\ to\ maternal\ conditions\ during\ a\ period \times 100,000}{Number\ of\ births\ during\ the\ period}$$

Vital Statistics Neonatal Mortality Rate (p. 86) [Chapter 6]

$$\frac{Number\ of\ neonatal\ deaths\ during\ a\ period \times 1,000}{Number\ of\ live\ births\ during\ the\ period}$$

World Health Organization formula for Maternal Mortality Rate (p. 85) [Chapter 6]

$$\frac{Number\ of\ maternal\ deaths \times 100,000}{Number\ of\ live\ births}$$

Formulas Listed by Chapter in Which They Appear

Chapter 2

Average (p. 20)
Rate (p. 19)

Chapter 3

Average Daily Inpatient Census (p. 38)
Average Daily Inpatient Census for a Patient Care Unit (p. 39)
Average Daily Newborn Census (p. 39)

Chapter 4

Bed Occupancy Ratio (p. 46)
Bed Turnover Rate, Direct Formula (p. 53)

Chapter 9 *(continued)*

Chapter 10

Appendix B
Glossary of Healthcare Services and Statistical Terms

Accuracy: A characteristic of data that are free from significant error, up to date, and representative of relevant facts

Adjusted hospital autopsy rate: The proportion of hospital autopsies performed following the deaths of patients whose bodies are available for autopsy

Admission date: In the home health prospective payment system, the date of first service; in the acute care prospective payment system, the year, month, and day of inpatient admission, beginning with a hospital's formal acceptance of a patient who is to receive healthcare services while receiving room, board, and continuous nursing services

Aggregate data: Data extracted from individual health records and combined to form de-identified information about groups of patients that can be compared and analyzed

Alternative hypothesis: A hypothesis that states that there is an association between independent and dependent variables

Ambulatory care: Preventive or corrective healthcare services provided on a nonresident basis in a provider's office, clinic setting, or hospital outpatient setting

Analysis of variance (ANOVA): Test used to assess the differences among more than two means

Ancillary service visit: The appearance of an outpatient in a unit of a hospital or outpatient facility to receive services, tests, or procedures that ordinarily are not counted as encounters for healthcare services

Ancillary services: Tests and procedures ordered by a physician to provide information for use in patient diagnosis or treatment

Anesthesia death rate: The ratio of deaths caused by anesthetic agents to the number of anesthetics administered during a specified period of time

Applied research: A type of research that focuses on the use of scientific theories to improve actual practice as in medical research applied to the treatment of patients

Arithmetic mean length of stay (AMLOS):   The average length of stay for all patients

Autopsy: The postmortem examination of the organs and tissues of a body to determine the cause of death or pathological conditions

Autopsy rate: The proportion or percentage of deaths in a healthcare organization that are followed by the performance of an autopsy

Available for hospital autopsy: A situation in which the required conditions have been met to allow an autopsy to be performed on a hospital patient who has died

Average: The value obtained by dividing the sum of a set of numbers by the number of values

Average daily inpatient census: The mean number of hospital inpatients present in the hospital each day for a given period of time

Average duration of hospitalization: *See* **average length of stay**

Average length of stay (ALOS):   The mean length of stay for hospital inpatients discharged during a given period of time

Bar chart: A graphic technique used to display frequency distributions of nominal or ordinal data that fall into categories; also called bar graph

Bar graph: *See* **bar chart**

Basic research: A type of research that focuses on the development and refinement of theories

Bed capacity: The number of beds that a facility has been designed and constructed to house

Bed complement: *See* **bed count**

Bed count: The number of inpatient beds set up and staffed for use on a given day; also called bed complement

Bed count day: A unit of measure that denotes the presence of one inpatient bed (either occupied or vacant) set up and staffed for use in one 24-hour period

Bed occupancy ratio: The proportion of beds occupied, defined as the ratio of inpatient service days to bed count days during a specified period of time

Bed size: The total number of inpatient beds for which a facility is equipped and staffed to provide patient care services

Bed turnover rate: The average number of times a bed changes occupants during a given period of time

Boarder: An individual such as a parent, caregiver, or other family member who receives lodging at a healthcare facility but is not a patient

Boarder baby: A newborn who remains in the nursery following discharge because the mother is still hospitalized, or a premature infant who no longer needs intensive care but remains for observation

Budget: A plan that converts the organization's goals and objectives into targets for revenue and spending

Calculation of inpatient service days: The measurement of the services received by all inpatients in one 24-hour period

Calculation of transfers: A medical care unit that shows transfers on and off the unit as subdivisions of patients admitted to and discharged from the unit

Cancer mortality rate: The proportion of patients who die from cancer

Capital budget: The allocation of resources for long-term investments and projects

Case fatality rate: The total number of deaths due to a specific illness during a given time period divided by the total number of cases during the same period

Case-mix index: The average relative weight of all cases treated at a given facility or by a given physician, which reflects the resource intensity or clinical severity of a specific group in relation to the other groups in the classification system

Categorical data: Four types of data (nominal, ordinal, interval, and ratio) that represent values or observations that can be sorted into a category; also called scales of measurement

Causal research: A type of conclusive research that tries to answer questions about what causes certain things to occur.

Cause-specific death rate: The total number of deaths due to a specific illness during a given time period divided by the estimated population for the same time period

Census: The number of inpatients present in a healthcare facility at any given time

Census day: *See* **inpatient service day**

Census statistics: Statistics that examine the number of patients being treated at specific times, the lengths of their stay, and the number of times a bed changes occupants

Census survey: A survey that collects data from all the members of a population

Centers for Disease Control and Prevention (CDC):   A group of federal agencies that oversees health promotion and disease control and prevention activities in the United States

Centers for Medicare and Medicaid Services (CMS):   The division of the Department of Health and Human Services that is responsible for developing healthcare policy in the United States and for administering the Medicare program and the federal portion of the Medicaid program; called the Health Care Financing Administration (HCFA) prior to 2001

Certificate of need: A state-directed program that requires healthcare facilities to submit detailed plans and justifications for the purchase of new equipment, new buildings, or new service offerings that cost in excess of a certain amount

Cesarean-section rate: The ratio of all Cesarean sections to the total number of deliveries, including Cesarean sections, during a specified period of time

Chi square: A test of significance, represented by χ^2, that deals with nominal data and frequencies, specifically data where the standard deviation and mean are not meaningful descriptions

Chronic: Of long duration

Clean surgical case: A surgical case in which no infection existed prior to surgery

Clinic outpatient: A patient who is admitted to a clinical service of a clinic or hospital for diagnosis or treatment on an ambulatory basis

Clinical research: A specialized area of research that primarily investigates the efficacy of preventive, diagnostic, and therapeutic procedures; also called medical research

Cluster sampling: The process of selecting subjects for a sample from each cluster within a population (for example, a family, school, or community)

Community-acquired infection: An infectious disease contracted as the result of exposure before or after a patient's period of hospitalization

Complete master census: A total census for a facility showing the names and locations of patients present in the hospital at a particular point in time

Complication: A medical condition that arises during an inpatient hospitalization (for example, a postoperative wound infection)

Conclusive research: A type of research performed in order to come to some sort of conclusion or help in decision making; includes descriptive research and causal research

Concomitant: Accessory; taking place at the same time

Confidence interval: A healthcare statistic that is calculated from the standard error of the mean, it is an estimate of the true limits within which the true population mean lies; the range of values that may reasonably contain the true population mean

Consultation: The response by one healthcare professional to another healthcare professional's request to provide recommendations and/or opinions regarding the care of a particular patient or resident

Consultation rate: The total number of hospital inpatients receiving consultations for a given period divided by the total number of discharges and deaths for the same period

Continuous data: Data that represent measurable quantities but are not restricted to certain specified values

Control group: A comparison study group whose members do not undergo the treatment under study

Convenience sampling: A sampling technique where the selection of units from the population is based on easy availability and/or accessibility

Coroner: A public officer whose principal duty is to inquire via an inquest into the cause of any death that there is reason to suppose is not due to natural causes

Coroner's case: A death that appears to be suspicious and requires action from the coroner to determine the cause of death

Correlational research: A design of research that determines the existence and degree of relationships among factors

Cost–benefit analysis: A process that uses quantitative techniques to evaluate and measure the benefit of providing products or services compared to the cost of providing them

Crude birth rate: The number of live births divided by the population at risk

Crude death rate: The total number of deaths in a given population for a given period of time divided by the estimated population for the same period of time

Daily census: The number of inpatients present at the census-taking time each day, plus any inpatients who were both admitted after the previous census-taking time and discharged before the next census-taking time

Daily inpatient census: The number of inpatients present at census-taking time each day, plus any inpatients who were both admitted and discharged after the census-taking time the previous day

Data: The dates, numbers, images, symbols, letters, and words that represent basic facts and observations about people, processes, measurements, and conditions

Data accuracy: The extent to which data are free of identifiable errors

Data collection: The process by which data are gathered

Date of encounter (outpatient and physician services): The year, month, and day of a visit or other healthcare encounter

Date of procedure (inpatient): The year, month, and day of each significant procedure

Date of service (DOS): The date a test, procedure, or service was rendered

Days of stay: *See* **length of stay**

Dead on arrival (DOA): The condition of a patient who arrives at a healthcare facility with no signs of life and who was pronounced dead by a physician

Death rate: The proportion of inpatient hospitalizations that end in death

Decile: The tenth equal part of a distribution

Decimal: Numbered or proceeding by tens; based on the number 10; expressed in or utilizing a decimal system, especially with a decimal point

Delivery: The process of delivering a liveborn infant or dead fetus (and placenta) by manual, instrumental, or surgical means

Denominator: The part of a fraction below the line signifying division that functions as the divisor of the numerator and, in fractions with 1 as the numerator, indicates into how many parts the unit is divided

Dependent variable: A measurable variable in a research study that depends on an independent variable

Descriptive research: A type of conclusive research that determines and reports the current status of topics and subjects

Descriptive statistics: Statistics that describe populations

Discharge date: The year, month, and day that an inpatient was formally released from the hospital and room, board, and continuous nursing services were terminated

Discharge days: *See* **length of stay** and **total length of stay**

Discharge diagnosis list: A complete set of discharge diagnoses applicable to a single patient episode, such as an inpatient hospitalization

Discharge transfer: The transfer of an inpatient to another healthcare institution at the time of discharge

Discrete data: Data that represent separate and distinct values or observations; that is, data that contain only finite numbers and have only specified values

Disposition: For outpatients, the healthcare practitioner's description of the patient's status at discharge (no follow-up planned, follow-up planned or scheduled, referred elsewhere, expired), for inpatients, a core health data element that identifies the circumstances under which the patient left the hospital (discharged alive, discharged to home or self-care, discharged and transferred to another short-term general hospital for inpatient care, discharged and transferred to a skilled nursing facility, discharged and transferred to an intermediate care facility, discharged and transferred to another type of institution for inpatient care or referred for outpatient services to another institution, discharged and transferred to home under care of an organized home health services organization, discharged and transferred to home under care of a home intravenous therapy provider, left against medical advice or discontinued care, expired, status not stated)

Duration of inpatient hospitalization: *See* **length of stay**

Early fetal death: The death of a product of human conception that is fewer than 20 weeks of gestation and 500 grams or less in weight before its complete expulsion or extraction from the mother

Electronic health record (EHR):   A computerized record of health information and associated processes; also called computer-based patient record

Electronic medical record (EMR):   A form of computer-based health record in which information is stored in whole files instead of by individual data elements

Electronic signature: Any representation of a signature in digital form, including an image of a handwritten signature; also, the authentication of a computer entry in a health record made by the individual making the entry

Emergency patient: A patient who is admitted to the emergency services department of a hospital for the diagnosis and treatment of a condition that requires immediate medical, dental, or allied health services in order to sustain life or to prevent critical consequences

Encounter: The direct personal contact between a patient and a physician or other person authorized by state licensure law and, if applicable, by medical staff bylaws to order or furnish healthcare services for the diagnosis or treatment of the patient

Episode of care: A period of relatively continuous medical care performed by healthcare professionals in relation to a particular clinical problem or situation

Ethnography: A method of observational research that investigates culture in naturalistic settings using both qualitative and quantitative approaches

Evaluation research: A design of research that examines the effectiveness of policies, programs, or organizations

Exacerbation: To make more violent, bitter, or severe

Experimental research: A research design used to establish cause and effect; also, a controlled investigation in which subjects are assigned randomly to groups that experience carefully controlled interventions that are manipulated by the experimenter according to a strict protocol; also called experimental study

Exploratory research: A research design used because a problem has not been clearly defined or its scope is unclear

Fetal autopsy rate: The number of autopsies performed on intermediate and late fetal deaths for a given time period divided by the total number of intermediate and late fetal deaths for the same time period

Fetal death: The death of a product of human conception before its complete expulsion or extraction from the mother regardless of the duration of the pregnancy; also called stillborn

Fetal death rate: A proportion that compares the number of intermediate and/or late fetal deaths to the total number of live births and intermediate or late fetal deaths during the same period of time

Fiscal year: Any consecutive 12-month period an organization uses as its accounting period

Fraction: One or more parts of a whole

Frequency distribution: A table or graph that displays the number of times (frequency) a particular observation occurs

Frequency distribution table: A table consisting of a set of classes or categories along with the numerical counts that correspond to nominal and ordinal data

Frequency polygon: A type of line graph that represents a frequency distribution

Full-time equivalent employees (FTEs):   The total number of workers, including part-time, in an area as the equivalent of full-time positions

Gender: The biological sex of the patient as recorded at the start of care

Graph: A graphic tool used to show numerical data in a pictorial representation

Gross autopsy rate: The number of inpatient autopsies conducted during a given time period divided by the total number of inpatient deaths for the same time period

Gross death rate: The number of inpatient deaths that occurred during a given time period divided by the total number of inpatient discharges, including deaths, for the same time period

Histogram: A graphic technique used to display the frequency distribution of continuous data (interval or ratio data) as either numbers or percentages in a series of bars

Historical research: A research design used to investigate past events

Home health (HH):   An umbrella term that refers to the medical and nonmedical services provided to patients and their families in their places of residence; also called home care

Home health agency (HHA):   A program or organization that provides a blend of home-based medical and social services to homebound patients and their families for the purpose of promoting, maintaining, or restoring health or of minimizing the effects of illness, injury, or disability

Hospice: An interdisciplinary program of palliative care and supportive services that addresses the physical, spiritual, social, and economic needs of terminally ill patients and their families

Hospice care: The medical care provided to persons with life expectancies of six months or less who elect to forgo standard treatment of their illness and to receive only palliative care

Hospital: A healthcare entity that has an organized medical staff and permanent facilities that include inpatient beds and continuous medical and nursing services and that provides diagnostic and therapeutic services for patients, as well as overnight accommodations and nutritional services

Hospital ambulatory care: All hospital-directed preventive, therapeutic, and rehabilitative services provided by physicians and their surrogates to patients who are not hospital inpatients

Hospital autopsy: A postmortem (after-death) examination performed on the body of a person who has at some time been a hospital patient by a hospital pathologist or a physician of the medical staff who has been delegated the responsibility

Hospital autopsy rate: The total number of autopsies performed by a hospital pathologist for a given time period divided by the number of deaths of hospital patients (inpatients and outpatients) whose bodies were available for autopsy for the same time period

Hospital death rate: The number of inpatient deaths for a given period of time divided by the total number of live discharges and deaths for the same time period

Hospital inpatient: A patient who is provided with room, board, and continuous general nursing services in an area of an acute care facility where patients generally stay at least overnight

Hospital inpatient autopsy: A postmortem (after-death) examination performed on the body of a patient who died during an inpatient hospitalization by a hospital pathologist or a physician of the medical staff who has been delegated the responsibility

Hospital inpatient beds: Accommodations with supporting services (such as food, laundry, and housekeeping) for hospital inpatients, excluding those for the newborn nursery, but including incubators and bassinets in nurseries for premature or sick newborn infants

Hospital live birth: In an inpatient facility, the complete expulsion or extraction of a product of human conception from the mother, regardless of the duration of pregnancy, which, after such expulsion or extraction, breathes or shows any other evidence of life, such as beating of the heart, pulsation of the umbilical cord, or definite movement of voluntary muscles

Hospital newborn bassinet: Accommodations including incubators and isolettes in the newborn nursery with supporting services (such as food, laundry, and housekeeping) for hospital newborn inpatients

Hospital newborn inpatient: A patient born in the hospital at the beginning of the current inpatient hospitalization

Hospital outpatient: A hospital patient who receives services in one or more of a hospital's facilities when he or she is not currently an inpatient or a home care patient

Hospital outpatient care unit: An organized unit of a hospital that provides facilities and medical services exclusively or primarily to patients who are generally ambulatory and who do not currently require or are not currently receiving services as an inpatient of the hospital

Hospital-acquired infection: *See* **nosocomial infection**

Hospitalization: The period during an individual's life when he or she is a patient in a single hospital without interruption except by possible intervening leaves of absence

Hybrid health record: A combination of paper and electronic records

Hypothesis: A statement that describes a research question in measurable terms

Iatrogenic: Induced inadvertently by a physician or surgeon or by medical treatment or diagnostic procedures

Incidence rate: A computation that compares the number of new cases of a specific disease for a given time period to the population at risk for the disease during the same time period

Individually identifiable health information: According to HIPAA privacy provisions, that information which specifically identifies the patient to whom the information relates, such as age, gender, date of birth, and address

Induced termination of pregnancy: The purposeful interruption of an intrauterine pregnancy that was not intended to produce a liveborn infant and that did not result in a live birth

Infant death: The death of a liveborn infant at any time from the moment of birth to the end of the first year of life (364 days, 23 hours, 59 minutes from the moment of birth)

Infant mortality rate: The number of deaths of individuals under one year of age during a given time period divided by the number of live births reported for the same time period

Infection rate: The ratio of all infections to the number of discharges, including deaths

Inferential statistics: Statistics that are used to make inferences from a smaller group of data to a large one

Information: Data that have been deliberately selected, processed, and organized to be useful

Inpatient: *See* **hospital inpatient**

Inpatient admission: An acute care facility's formal acceptance of a patient who is to be provided with room, board, and continuous nursing service in an area of the facility where patients generally stay at least overnight

Inpatient bed count: *See* **bed count**

Inpatient bed occupancy rate: The total number of inpatient service days for a given time period divided by the total number of inpatient bed count days for the same time period; also called percentage of occupancy

Inpatient census: *See* **census**

Inpatient days of stay: *See* **length of stay**

Inpatient discharge: The termination of hospitalization through the formal release of an inpatient from a hospital

Inpatient service day: A unit of measure equivalent to the services received by one inpatient during one 24-hour period

Institutional death rate: *See* **net death rate**

Institutional Review Board (IRB):   An administrative body that provides oversight for the research studies conducted within a healthcare institution

Instrument: A standardized and uniform way to collect data

Intermediate fetal death: The death of a product of human conception before its complete expulsion or extraction from the mother that has completed 20 weeks of gestation (but less than 28 weeks) and weighs 501 to 1,000 grams

Internal validity: An attribute of a study's design that contributes to the accuracy of its findings

Interval data: A type of data that represents observations that can be measured on an evenly distributed scale beginning at a point other than true zero

Interview guide: A list of written questions to be asked during an interview

Intrahospital transfer: A change in medical care unit, medical staff unit, or responsible physician during hospitalization

Intrarater reliability: A measure of a research instrument's reliability in which the same person repeating the test will get reasonably similar findings

Judgment sampling: A sampling technique where the researcher relies on his or her own judgment to select the subjects

Knowledge: The information, understanding, and experience that give individuals the power to make informed decisions

Late fetal death: The death of a product of human conception that is 28 weeks or more of gestation and weighs 1,001 grams or more before its complete expulsion or extraction from the mother

Leave of absence: The authorized absence of an inpatient from a hospital or other facility for a specified period of time occurring after admission and prior to discharge

Leave of absence day: A day occurring after the admission and prior to the discharge of a hospital inpatient when the patient is not present at the census-taking hour because he or she is on leave of absence from the healthcare facility

Length of stay (LOS):   The total number of patient days for an inpatient episode, calculated by subtracting the date of admission from the date of discharge

Line graph: A graphic technique used to illustrate the relationship between continuous measurements; consists of a line drawn to connect a series of points on an arithmetic scale and is often used to display time trends

Literature review: A systematic investigation of all the knowledge available about a topic from sources such as books, journal articles, theses, and dissertations

Low-birth-weight neonate: Any newborn baby, regardless of gestational age, whose weight at birth is less than 2,500 grams

Managed care: A generic term for reimbursement and delivery systems that integrate the financing and provision of healthcare services by means of entering contractual agreements with selected providers to furnish comprehensive healthcare services and developing explicit criteria for the selection of healthcare providers, formal programs of ongoing quality improvement and utilization review, and significant financial incentives for members to use providers associated with the plan

Managed care organization (MCO): A type of healthcare organization that delivers medical care and manages all aspects of the care or the payment for care by limiting providers of care, discounting payment to providers of care, or limiting access to care

Maternal death: The death of any woman, from any cause, related to or aggravated by pregnancy or its management (regardless of duration or site of pregnancy), but not from accidental or incidental causes

Maternal death rate: For a hospital, the total number of maternal deaths directly related to pregnancy for a given time period divided by the total number of obstetrical discharges for the same time period; for a community, the total number of deaths attributed to maternal conditions during a given time period in a specific geographic area divided by the total number of live births for the same time period in the same area

Mean: A measure of central tendency that is determined by calculating the arithmetic average of the observations in a frequency distribution

Measure: A term referring to the quantifiable data about a function or process

Measurement: The systematic process of data collection, repeated over time or at a single point in time

Measures of central tendency: The typical or average numbers that are descriptive of the entire collection of data for a specific population

Median: A measure of central tendency that shows the midpoint of a frequency distribution when the observations have been arranged in order from lowest to highest

Medical examiner: *See* **coroner**

Medical services: The activities relating to medical care performed by physicians, nurses, and other healthcare professional and technical personnel under the direction of a physician

Method: A way of performing an action or task; also, a strategy used by a researcher to collect, analyze, and present data

Military time: Time measured in hours numbered to 24 (as 0100 or 2300) from one midnight to the next

Mode: A measure of central tendency that consists of the most frequent observation in a frequency distribution

Morbidity: A term referring to the state of being diseased (including illness, injury, or deviation from normal health); the number of sick persons or cases of disease in relationship to a specific population

Morgue: The place where the bodies of persons who have died are kept until identified and claimed by relatives or released for burial

Mortality: A term referring to the incidence of death in a specific population; also, the loss of subjects during the course of a clinical research study, or attrition

Mortality rate: A rate that measures the risk of death for the cause under study in a defined population during a given time period

Multivariate: In reference to research studies, a term meaning that many variables were involved

Naturalistic observation: A type of nonparticipant observation in which researchers observe certain behaviors and events as they occur naturally

Necropsy: *See* **autopsy**

Neonatal death: The death of a liveborn infant within the first 27 days, 23 hours, and 59 minutes following the moment of birth

Neonatal mortality rate: The number of deaths of infants under 28 days of age during a given time period divided by the total number of births for the same time period

Neonatal period: The period of an infant's life from the hour of birth through the first 27 days, 23 hours, and 59 minutes of life

Net autopsy rate: The ratio of inpatient autopsies compared to inpatient deaths calculated by dividing the total number of inpatient autopsies performed by the hospital pathologist for a given time period by the total number of inpatient deaths minus unautopsied coroners' or medical examiners' cases for the same time period

Net death rate: The total number of inpatient deaths minus the number of deaths that occurred less than 48 hours after admission for a given time period divided by the total number of inpatient discharges minus the number of deaths that occurred less than 48 hours after admission for the same time period

Newborn (NB):   An inpatient who was born in a hospital at the beginning of the current inpatient hospitalization

Newborn autopsy rate: The number of autopsies performed on newborns who died during a given time period divided by the total number of newborns who died during the same time period

Newborn bassinet count: The number of available hospital newborn bassinets, both occupied and vacant, on any given day

Newborn bassinet count day: A unit of measure that denotes the presence of one newborn bassinet, either occupied or vacant, set up and staffed for use in one 24-hour period

Newborn death: The death of a liveborn infant born in the hospital who later dies during the same admission

Newborn death rate: The number of newborns who died divided by the total number of newborns, both alive and dead; also called newborn mortality rate

Newborn mortality rate: The number of newborns who died divided by the total number of newborns, both alive and dead

Nominal data: A type of data that represents values or observations that can be labeled or named and where the values fall into unordered categories; also called dichotomous data

Normal distribution of data: A continuous frequency distribution characterized by a bell-shaped curve; that is, the mean, median, and mode are equal and most of the measurements are near the center of the frequency

Nosocomial infection: An infection acquired by a patient while receiving care or services in a healthcare organization; also called hospital-acquired infection

Nosocomial infection rate: The number of hospital-acquired infections for a given time period divided by the total number of inpatient discharges for the same time period

Null hypothesis: A hypothesis that states there is no association between the independent and dependent variables in a research study

Numerator: The part of a fraction that is above the line and signifies the number of parts of the denominator taken

Numerical data: Data that include discrete data and continuous data

Nursing facility: A comprehensive term for long-term care facilities that provide nursing care and related services on a 24-hour basis for residents requiring medical, nursing, or rehabilitative care

Observation: Service in which providers observe and monitor a patient to decide whether the patient needs to be admitted to inpatient care or can be discharged to home or outpatient area, usually charged by the hour

Observation patient: A patient who presents with a medical condition with a significant degree of instability and disability and who needs to be monitored, evaluated, and assessed to determine whether he or she should be admitted for inpatient care or discharged for care in another setting

Occasion of service: A specified, identifiable service that involves the care of a patient but is not an encounter (for example, a lab test ordered during an encounter)

Occupancy percent/ratio: *See* **bed occupancy ratio**

Operation: *See* **surgical operation**

Operational budget: A type of budget that allocates and controls resources to meet an organization's goals and objectives for the fiscal year

Ordinal data: A type of data that represents values or observations that can be ranked or ordered

Outlier: An extreme statistical value that falls outside the normal range

Outpatient: A patient who receives ambulatory care services in a hospital-based clinic or department

Patient: A living or deceased individual who is receiving or has received healthcare services

Patient care unit (PCU): An organizational entity of a healthcare facility organized both physically and functionally to provide care

Patient day: *See* **inpatient service day**

Payback period: A financial method used to evaluate the value of a capital expenditure by calculating the time frame that must pass before inflow of cash from a project equals or exceeds outflow of cash

Percentage: A value computed on the basis of the whole divided into 100 parts

Percent/percentage of occupancy: *See* **inpatient bed occupancy rate**

Perinatal death: An all-inclusive term that refers to both stillborn infants and neonatal deaths

Pictogram: A graphic technique in which pictures are used in the display of data

Pie chart: A graphic technique in which the proportions of a category are displayed as portions of a circle (like pieces of a pie)

Pie graph: *See* **pie chart**

Population: The universe of data under investigation from which a sample is taken

Postmortem examination: *See* **autopsy**

Postneonatal death: The death of a liveborn infant from 28 days to the end of the first year of life (364 days, 23 hours, and 59 minutes from the moment of birth)

Postneonatal mortality rate: The number of deaths of persons aged 28 days up to, but not including, one year during a given time period divided by the number of live births for the same time period

Postoperative death rate: The ratio of deaths within 10 days after surgery to the total number of operations performed during a specified period of time

Postoperative infection rate: The number of infections that occur in clean surgical cases for a given time period divided by the total number of operations within the same time period

Postpartum: Occurring after childbirth

Postterm neonate: Any neonate whose birth occurs from the beginning of the first day of the 43rd week (295th day) following onset of the last menstrual period

Pre-existing condition: Any injury, disease, or physical condition occurring prior to an arbitrary date

Prepartum: Occurring prior to childbirth

Preterm infant: An infant with a birth weight between 1,000 and 2,499 grams and/or a gestation between 28 and 37 completed weeks

Preterm neonate: Any neonate whose birth occurs through the end of the last day of the 38th week (266th day) following onset of the last menstrual period

Primary data source: Record developed by healthcare professionals in the process of providing patient care

Primary research: Data collected specifically for a study

Procedure: *See* **surgical procedure**

Productivity: A unit of performance defined by management in quantitative standards

Profiling: A measurement of the quality, utilization, and cost of medical resources provided by physicians that is made by employers, third-party payers, government entities, and other purchasers of healthcare

Proportion: The relation of one part to another or to the whole with respect to magnitude, quantity, or degree

Puerperal: The period immediately following childbirth

Qualitative research: A philosophy of research that assumes that multiple contextual truths exist and bias is always present; also called naturalism

Quantitative research: A philosophy of research that assumes that there is a single truth across time and place and that researchers are able to adopt a neutral, unbiased stance and establish causation; also called positivism

Quartile: The fourth equal part of a distribution

Questionnaire: A type of survey in which the members of the population are questioned through the use of electronic or paper forms

Quota sampling: A sampling technique where the population is first segmented into mutually exclusive subgroups, just as in stratified sampling, and then judgment is used to select the subjects or units from each segment based on a specified proportion

Quotient: The number resulting from the division of one number by another

Random sampling: An unbiased selection of subjects that includes methods such as simple random sampling, stratified random sampling, systematic sampling, and cluster sampling

Randomization: The assignment of subjects to experimental or control groups based on chance

Range: Distance or extent between possible extremes

Ranked data: A type of ordinal data where the observations are first arranged from highest to lowest according to magnitude and then assigned numbers that correspond to each observation's place in the sequence

Rate: A measure used to compare an event over time; a comparison of the number of times an event did happen (numerator) with the number of times an event could have happened (denominator)

Ratio: A calculation found by dividing one quantity by another; also, a general term that can include a number of specific measures such as proportion, percentage, and rate

Ratio data: Data that may be displayed by units of equal size and placed on a scale starting with zero and thus can be manipulated mathematically (for example, 0, 5, 10, 15, 20)

Recap: Abbreviation of *recapitulation*

Recapitulation: A concise summary of data

Recurrence: To occur again after an interval

Relevance: How applicable information is to some matter

Reliability: A measure of consistency of data items based on their reproducibility and an estimation of their error of measurement

Research: Investigation or experimentation aimed at the discovery and interpretation of facts, revision of accepted theories or laws in the light of new facts, or practical application of such new or revised theories or laws; the collecting of information about a particular subject

Research data: Data used for the purpose of answering a proposed question or testing a hypothesis

Return on investment (ROI):   The financial analysis of the extent of value a major purchase will provide

Rounding: The process of approximating a number

Run chart: A type of graph that shows data points collected over time and identifies emerging trends or patterns

Sample: A set of units selected for study that represents a population

Sample size: The number of subjects needed in a study to represent a population

Sample size calculation: The qualitative and quantitative procedures to determine an appropriate sample size

Sample survey: A type of survey that collects data from representative members of a population

Scales of measurement: *See* **categorical data**

Scatter diagram: A graph that visually displays the linear relationships among factors

Secondary data source: Data derived from the primary patient record, such as an index or database

Secondary record: A record derived from the primary record and containing selected data elements

Secondary research: Data collected from a literature review

Skewness: The horizontal stretching of a frequency distribution to one side or the other so that one tail is longer than the other

Spreadsheet: Worksheet into which text, numbers, and formulas are entered to assist with calculations

Standard error of the mean: A value that is found by taking many large samples, calculating the mean for each sample, and then finding the standard deviation of all the sample means

Standard deviation: A measure of variability that describes the deviation from the mean of a frequency distribution in the original units of measurement; the square root of the variance

Statistics: A branch of mathematics concerned with collecting, organizing, summarizing, and analyzing data

Stillbirth: The birth of a fetus, regardless of gestational age, that shows no evidence of life (such as heartbeats or respirations) after complete expulsion or extraction from the mother during childbirth

Stratified random sampling: The process of selecting the same percentages of subjects for a study sample as they exist in the subgroups (strata) of the population

Structured interview: An interview format that uses a set of standardized questions that are asked of all applicants

Surgical death rate: *See* **postoperative death rate**

Surgical operation: One or more surgical procedures performed at one time for one patient via a common approach or for a common purpose

Surgical procedure: Any single, separate, systematic process upon or within the body that can be complete in itself; is normally performed by a physician, dentist, or other licensed practitioner; can be performed with or without instruments; and is performed to restore disunited or deficient parts, remove diseased or injured tissues, extract foreign matter, assist in obstetrical delivery, or aid in diagnosis

Survey: A type of research instrument with which the members of the population being studied are asked questions and respond orally

Systematic random sampling: The process of selecting a sample of subjects for a study by drawing every *n*th unit on a list

t **test:**   A test of the null hypothesis to determine if a set of results is statistically significant.

Table: An organized arrangement of data, usually in columns and rows

Term neonate: Any neonate whose birth occurs from the beginning of the first day of the 39th week (267th day) through the end of the last day of the 42nd week (294th day) following onset of the last menstrual period

Total bed count days: The sum of inpatient bed count days for each of the days during a specified period of time

Total discharge days: *See* **total length of stay**

Total inpatient service days: The sum of all inpatient service days for each of the days during a specified period of time

Total length of stay: The sum of the days of stay of any group of inpatients discharged during a specific period of time; also called discharge days

Transfer: The movement of a patient from one treatment service or location to another; *see also* **intrahospital transfer**

Type I error: Occurs when the null hypothesis is rejected, yet it is actually true

Type II error: Occurs when the null hypothesis is not rejected, yet it is false

Unit labor cost: Cost determined by dividing the total annual compensation by total annual productivity

Unrestricted question: A type of question that allows free-form responses; also called open-ended question

Utilization management: A program that evaluates the healthcare facility's efficiency in providing necessary care to patients in the most effective manner

Validity: The extent to which data correspond to the actual state of affairs or that an instrument measures what it purports to measure; also, a term referring to a test's ability to accurately and consistently measure what it purports to measure

Variability: The difference between each score and every other score in a frequency distribution

Variable: A characteristic or property that may take on different values

Variance: A disagreement between two parts; the square of the standard deviation

Variance analysis: An assessment of a department's financial transactions to identify differences between the budget amount and the actual amount of a line item

Visit: A single encounter with a healthcare professional that includes all the services supplied during the encounter

Vital statistics: Data related to births, deaths, marriages, and fetal deaths

Well newborn: A newborn born at term, under sterile conditions, with no diseases, conditions, disorders, syndromes, injuries, malformations, or defects diagnosed, and no operations other than routine circumcision performed

Whole number: Any of the set of nonnegative integers

World Health Organization (WHO):   The United Nations specialized agency created to ensure the attainment by all peoples of the highest possible levels of health and responsible for a number of international classifications, including *The International Statistical Classification of Diseases & Related Health Problems* (ICD-10) and *The International Classification of Functioning, Disability & Health* (ICF)

Appendix C
Answers to Odd-Numbered Chapter Exercises

Chapter 1

Exercise 1.1

Identify the following as either a Primary Data Source or a Secondary Data Source:

1. Health insurance data pulled from national census	**Secondary**
2. Hospital census	**Primary**
3. Productivity reports pulled from patient visit report	**Secondary**
4. Patient health record	**Primary**
5. State vital statistics	**Primary**
6. Tumor registry	**Secondary**
7. Hospital disease index	**Secondary**

Chapter 2

Exercise 2.1

1. $\dfrac{40}{80} = \dfrac{4}{8} = \dfrac{1}{2}$

2. $\dfrac{3}{9} = \dfrac{1}{3}$

3. $\dfrac{75}{150} = \dfrac{1}{2}$

4. $\dfrac{6}{36} = \dfrac{1}{6}$

5. $\dfrac{20}{100} = \dfrac{2}{10} = \dfrac{1}{5}$

Exercise 2.3

1. 48 = 50
2. 356 = 360
3. 311 = 310
4. 5,896 = 5,900
5. 3,258 = 3,260
6. 9,631 = 9,630
7. 232,563 = 232,560
8. 2,634 = 2,630
9. 48,605 = 48,610
10. 8,563 = 8,560
11. 651 = 700
12. 123 = 100
13. 8,307 = 8,300
14. 7,534 = 7,500
15. 5,781 = 5,800
16. 18.3 = 18
17. 32.5 = 33
18. 23.1 = 23
19. 152.6 = 153
20. 99.4 = 99
21. 15.89 = 15.9
22. 18.58 = 18.6
23. 32.62 = 32.6
24. 99.98 = 100.0
25. 124.07 = 124.1
26. 7.897438 = 7.90
27. 12.14526 = 12.15
28. 0.569888 = 0.57
29. 27.99999 = 28.00

Exercise 2.5

1. Sickle-cell: $\dfrac{1}{2}$

   Hemophilia: $\dfrac{3}{10}$

   Ewing's sarcoma: $\dfrac{3}{20}$

   Wilms' tumor: $\dfrac{1}{20}$

2. Sickle-cell: 0.5

   Hemophilia: 0.3

   Ewing's sarcoma: 0.15

   Wilms' tumor: 0.05

3. Sickle-cell: 50%

   Hemophilia: 30%

   Ewing's sarcoma: 15%

   Wilms' tumor: 5%

Exercise 2.7

1. $\dfrac{15}{(435+15)} = 0.03$

2. $\dfrac{12}{(12+38)} = 0.24$

Chapter 3

Exercise 3.1

1. Yes. The counts could have differed. Any number of admissions, discharges, or transfers could have occurred between 12 midnight and 1 a.m. on either day.

2. No. The total hospital census would be inconsistent. Every PCU in the hospital should follow the same administrative procedures.

3. No. The patient cannot be in two places at the same time. If both units are counting heads only once a day at midnight, the patient is counted as being present in unit A only. However, the patient is indicated in unit B's census as a transfer.

Exercise 3.3

Compare the definition of inpatient service day to the definitions of daily inpatient census and inpatient census. Will the figure representing an inpatient service day for any one day be the same as the figure for a daily inpatient census or inpatient census?

It will be the same as the figure for the daily inpatient census. (It can be the same as the inpatient census, provided there were no patients admitted/discharged on the same day.)

Exercise 3.5

1. c. Both a and b

2. c. Total inpatient service days

3. b. Consistent

4. a. Counted where he or she is

5. a. Inpatient service day

6. d. 59

7. a. Inpatient census: The number of inpatients present in a healthcare facility at any given time

   b. Daily inpatient census: The number of inpatients present at the census-taking time each day, plus any inpatients who were both admitted after the previous census-taking time and discharged before the next census-taking time

   c. Inpatient service day: A unit of measure equivalent to the services received by one inpatient during one 24-hour period

   d. Total inpatient service days: The sum of all inpatient service days for each of the days during a specified period of time

Exercise 3.7

Day	12:01 a.m. Census A/C	NB	Adm A/C	Bir	Trf in	Total A/C	NB	Dis A/C	Dis NB	Trf out	11:59 p.m. Census A/C	NB	A/D	Serv Days A/C	NB
6/1	250	18	20	4	2	**272**	**22**	25	3	2	**245**	**19**	1	**246**	**19**
6/2	**245**	**19**	22	6	1	**268**	**25**	24	5	1	**243**	**20**	0	**243**	**20**
6/3	**243**	**20**	24	5	0	**267**	**25**	23	4	0	**244**	**21**	3	**247**	**21**
6/4	**244**	**21**	22	3	1	**267**	**24**	22	3	1	**244**	**21**	1	**245**	**21**
6/5	**244**	**21**	25	4	2	**271**	**25**	25	3	2	**244**	**22**	2	**246**	**22**

Exercise 3.9

Worksheet No. 1

Monthly Compilation of Inpatient Census and Inpatient Service Days May 20XX															
Day	12:01 a.m. Census A/C	NB	Adm A/C	Bir	Trf in	Total A/C	NB	Dis A/C	NB	Trf out	11:59 p.m. Census A/C	NB	A/D	Serv Days A/C	NB
1	162	2	22	1	10	194	3	19	0	10	165	3	1	166	3
2	165	3	29	0	8	**202**	**3**	23	1	8	**171**	**2**	0	**171**	**2**
3	**171**	**2**	14	2	3	**188**	**4**	24	0	3	**161**	**4**	1	**162**	**4**

Monthly Compilation of Inpatient Census and Inpatient Service Days May 20XX														
	12:01 a.m. Census		Adm		Trf	Total		Dis		Trf	11:59 p.m. Census			Serv Days	
Day	A/C	NB	A/C	Bir	in	A/C	NB	A/C	NB	out	A/C	NB	A/D	A/C	NB
4	161	4	24	0	5	190	4	25	0	5	160	4	0	160	4
5	160	4	11	1	6	177	5	25	2	6	146	3	0	146	3
6	146	3	20	0	1	167	3	16	0	1	150	3	0	150	3
7	150	3	29	0	10	189	3	17	0	10	162	3	0	162	3
8	162	3	24	2	13	199	5	20	0	13	166	5	3	169	5
9	166	5	23	1	7	196	6	22	1	7	167	5	1	168	5
10	167	5	19	0	10	196	5	17	0	10	169	5	0	169	5
11	169	5	11	0	5	185	5	22	3	5	158	2	1	159	2
12	158	2	16	0	6	180	2	24	0	6	150	2	0	150	2
13	150	2	18	1	5	173	3	25	0	5	143	3	0	143	3
14	143	3	29	0	5	177	3	19	0	5	153	3	0	153	3
15	153	3	28	0	8	189	3	22	2	8	159	1	1	160	1
16	159	1	26	3	6	191	4	19	0	6	166	4	0	166	4
17	166	4	26	0	7	199	4	19	2	7	173	2	0	173	2
18	173	2	18	0	10	201	2	25	0	10	166	2	0	166	2
19	166	2	12	0	6	184	2	33	0	6	145	2	0	145	2
20	145	2	22	1	8	175	3	16	3	8	151	0	1	152	0
21	151	0	26	0	3	180	0	17	0	3	160	0	1	161	0
22	160	0	32	2	11	203	2	25	0	11	167	2	1	168	2
23	167	2	29	2	14	210	4	27	0	14	169	4	0	169	4
24	169	4	22	0	10	201	4	21	2	10	170	2	0	170	2
25	170	2	20	3	13	203	5	34	0	13	156	5	0	156	5
26	156	5	14	0	6	176	5	37	1	6	133	4	1	134	4
27	133	4	23	0	5	161	4	16	0	5	140	4	0	140	4
28	140	4	26	2	4	170	6	18	2	4	148	4	0	148	4
29	148	4	17	0	6	171	4	22	1	6	143	3	1	144	3
30	143	3	19	0	7	169	3	21	1	7	141	2	0	141	2
31	141	2	21	1	12	174	3	16	0	12	146	3	1	147	3
Total			670	22				686	21				14	4,868	91

Exercise 3.9 (*continued*)

Worksheet No. 2

Recap of Monthly Data for Adults and Children: May 20XX
(enter numbers from Worksheet No. 1)

12:01 a.m. Census A/C		162
Adm A/C	+	**670**
Trf in	+	**230**
Total A/C	=	**1,062**
Dis A/C	−	**686**
Trf out	−	**230**
11:59 p.m. Census A/C	=	146

Recap of Monthly Data for Newborns:

12:01 a.m. Census NB		2
Bir	+	**22**
Total NB	=	**24**
Dis NB	−	**21**
11:59 p.m. Census NB	=	3

Serv days A/C (total inpatient service days excluding newborns): **4,868**

Serv days NB (total newborn service days): **91**

Total inpatient service days: 4,959

Chapter 4

Exercise 4.1

   No.

Exercise 4.3

Children's Hospital
April 20XX

Unit	Bed Count	Inpatient Service Days	Percentage of Occupancy
Pediatric Medicine	55	1,450	$\dfrac{(1,450 \times 100)}{(55 \times 30)} = 87.9\%$
Pediatric Surgery	40	1,059	$\dfrac{(1,059 \times 100)}{(40 \times 30)} = 88.3\%$
Respiratory	25	642	$\dfrac{(642 \times 100)}{(25 \times 30)} = 85.6\%$
Hematology/Oncology	38	1,122	$\dfrac{(1,122 \times 100)}{(38 \times 30)} = 98.4\%$
Pediatric ICU	12	275	$\dfrac{(275 \times 100)}{(12 \times 30)} = 76.4\%$
Pediatric Cardiac ICU	10	261	$\dfrac{(261 \times 100)}{(10 \times 30)} = 87.0\%$
Neonatal ICU	20	456	$\dfrac{(456 \times 100)}{(20 \times 30)} = 76.0\%$
Total	**200**	**5,265**	

$$\textbf{TOTAL PERCENTAGE OF OCCUPANCY} = \frac{(5,265 \times 100)}{(200 \times 30)} = \frac{526,500}{6,000} = 87.75 = 87.8\%$$

Exercise 4.5

Community Hospital
December 20XX

PCU	Inpatient Service Days	Bed Count	Percentage of Occupancy
Med/Surg	1,876	70	$\dfrac{(1,876 \times 100)}{(70 \times 31)} = \dfrac{187,600}{2,170} = 86.45 = 86.5\%$
ICU	300	10	$\dfrac{(300 \times 100)}{(10 \times 31)} = \dfrac{30,000}{310} = 96.77 = 96.8\%$
CCU	240	8	$\dfrac{(240 \times 100)}{(8 \times 31)} = \dfrac{24,000}{248} = 96.77 = 96.8\%$
Rehabilitation	300	12	$\dfrac{(300 \times 100)}{(12 \times 31)} = \dfrac{30,000}{372} = 80.6\%$
Burn	75	5	$\dfrac{(75 \times 100)}{(5 \times 31)} = \dfrac{7,500}{155} = 48.38 = 48.4\%$
Psychiatry	200	15	$\dfrac{(200 \times 100)}{(15 \times 31)} = \dfrac{20,000}{465} = 43.0\%$
Pediatric	870	30	$\dfrac{(870 \times 100)}{(30 \times 31)} = \dfrac{87,000}{930} = 93.5\%$
Total	**3,861**	**150**	$\dfrac{(3,861 \times 100)}{(150 \times 31)} = \dfrac{386,100}{4,650} = 83.0\%$
Nursery	280	10	$\dfrac{(280 \times 100)}{(10 \times 31)} = \dfrac{28,000}{310} = 90.3\%$

Exercise 4.7

1. Turnover rate (direct formula): $\dfrac{6{,}500}{200} = 32.5$

2. Turnover rate (indirect formula): $\dfrac{(0.8 \times 365)}{9} = \dfrac{292}{9} = 32.4$

Chapter 5

Exercise 5.1

Calculate the LOS for the following discharged patients in an acute care facility.

Date Admitted	Date Discharged	Length of Stay
5/3	5/4	**1**
7/2	7/12	**10**
2/14	2/28	**14**
3/25	4/15	**21**
8/27	9/10	**14**

Exercise 5.3

1. Calculate the time it takes to see patients in this physician's office.

Time Admitted	Time Seen by Physician	Time between Checking In at Reception and Being Seen by Physician
8:00 a.m.	8:17 a.m.	**17 minutes**
1:22 p.m.	2:05 p.m.	**43 minutes**
10:30 a.m.	11:43 a.m.	**73 minutes**

For example, 11:43 – 11:00 = 43 minutes. 11:00 – 10:30 = 30 minutes. 43 + 30 = 73 minutes.

2. a.

Patient 02.04.2012	Time of Arrival (Time "A")	Time Patient Was Triaged (Time "B")	Wait Time
Patient A	8:00	8:18	**18 minutes**
Patient B	8:30	8:55	**25 minutes**
Patient C	9:26	10:47	**1 hour 21 minutes**
Patient D	10:02	1:25	**3 hours 23 minutes**
Patient E	11:45	2:04	**2 hours 19 minutes**
Patient F	1:15	1:59	**44 minutes**
Patient G	2:30	3:10	**40 minutes**
Patient H	2:45	3:50	**1 hour 5 minutes**

b. **Average wait time: 77 minutes or 1 hour and 17 minutes**

c. **NO**, the hospital ER is not in compliance.

Exercise 5.5

1. $\dfrac{825}{158} = 5.2$ days

2. True

3.

University Hospital
May 20XX

Clinical Units	Discharges	Discharge Days	ALOS
Surgery	1,720	8,627	$\dfrac{8,627}{1,720} = 5.0$
Medicine	1,594	7,852	$\dfrac{7,852}{1,594} = 4.9$
Neurology	988	4,285	$\dfrac{4,285}{988} = 4.3$
Oncology	878	18,588	$\dfrac{18,588}{878} = 21.2$
Obstetrics/Gynecology	588	1,479	$\dfrac{1,479}{588} = 2.5$
Ophthalmology	385	1,154	$\dfrac{1,154}{385} = 3.0$
Orthopedics	651	9,321	$\dfrac{9,321}{651} = 14.3$
Pediatrics	358	2,841	$\dfrac{2,841}{358} = 7.9$
Psychiatry	156	4,697	$\dfrac{4,697}{156} = 30.1$
Rehabilitation	321	8,057	$\dfrac{8,057}{321} = 25.1$
Urology	89	183	$\dfrac{183}{89} = 2.1$
Total	**7,728**	**67,084**	$\dfrac{67,084}{7,728} = 8.7$

Exercise 5.7

1.

Admitted	Discharged	LOS
1/12	1/31	**19**
7/4	7/30	**26**
01/01/2008 (2008 is a leap year)	2/1/2009	**397**
11/24	11/24	**1**
6/19/2007	1/4/2009	**565**

2. $19 + 26 + 397 + 1 + 565 = 1{,}008$ days

3. $\dfrac{92{,}725}{15{,}987} = 5.8$ days

4. $\dfrac{11{,}062}{3{,}421} = 3.2$ days

5. $\dfrac{51{,}201}{11{,}644} = 4.4$ days

6. $\dfrac{32{,}103}{4{,}852} = 6.6$ days

7. $\dfrac{10{,}483}{2{,}912} = 3.6$ days

8.

Community Hospital
Medicare Discharge Statistics
July 20XX

Unit	Medicare Discharges	Medicare Discharge Days	ALOS
Medicine	325	2,375	$\dfrac{\mathbf{2{,}375}}{\mathbf{325}} = \mathbf{7.3}$
Surgery	175	2,103	$\dfrac{\mathbf{2{,}103}}{\mathbf{175}} = \mathbf{12.0}$
Rehabilitation	298	4,179	$\dfrac{\mathbf{4{,}179}}{\mathbf{298}} = \mathbf{14.0}$
Skilled Nursing	305	6,588	$\dfrac{\mathbf{6{,}588}}{\mathbf{305}} = \mathbf{21.6}$

Chapter 6

Exercise 6.1
1.63%
Total the deaths of adults, children, and newborns and multiply that by 100—then divide by the total discharges of adults, children, and newborns. In this case the deaths have to be added into the discharges in the denominator.

$$\frac{(9+1)\times100}{(540+62)+(9+1)}=\frac{1,000}{612}=1.63\%$$

Exercise 6.3
Net death rate:

$$\frac{[(5\ A\&C\ deaths+2\ NB\ deaths)-(1\ A\&C\ death<48\ hours+1\ NB\ death<48\ hours)\times100]}{(307\ A\&C\ discharges+5\ A\&C\ deaths)+(62\ NB\ discharges+2\ NB\ deaths)-(1\ A\&C\ death<48\ hours+1\ NB\ death<48\ hours)}=\frac{(7-2)\times100}{(312+64-2)}=\frac{500}{374}=1.34\%$$

Exercise 6.5

Community Hospital
January–March 20XX
Number of Surgery Patients and Deaths, by Surgeon

Physician Number	No. of Surgery Patients	No. of Deaths within 10 Days after Surgery	Postoperative Death Rate
Dr. 102	180	4	$\frac{(4\times100)}{180}=2.22\%$
Dr. 237	120	2	$\frac{(2\times100)}{120}=1.67\%$
Dr. 391	60	1	$\frac{(1\times100)}{60}=1.67\%$
Dr. 518	65	1	$\frac{(1\times100)}{65}=1.54\%$
Dr. 637	98	5	$\frac{(5\times100)}{98}=5.10\%$
Dr. 802	32	3	$\frac{(3\times100)}{32}=9.38\%$
Dr. 900	64	1	$\frac{(1\times100)}{64}=1.56\%$

Exercise 6.7

**Community Hospital
July–December 20XX
Selected MS-DRGs—Postoperative Deaths
Number of Surgery Patients and Deaths
Surgery Service**

MS-DRG	MS-DRG Title	No. of Surgery Patients	No. of Deaths within 10 Days after Surgery	Postoperative Death Rate
338	Appendectomy w complicated principal diag w MCC	8	1	$\dfrac{(1\times100)}{8}=12.50\%$
327	Stomach, esophageal & duodenal proc w CC	67	2	$\dfrac{(2\times100)}{67}=2.99\%$
005	Liver transplant w MCC or intestinal transplant	17	6	$\dfrac{(6\times100)}{17}=35.29\%$
139	Salivary gland procedures	5	1	$\dfrac{(1\times100)}{5}=20.00\%$
405	Pancreas, liver & shunt procedures w MCC	54	3	$\dfrac{(3\times100)}{54}=5.56\%$
625	Thyroid, parathyroid & thyroglossal procedures w MCC	195	2	$\dfrac{(2\times100)}{195}=1.03\%$
736	Uterine & adnexa proc for ovarian or adnexal malignancy w MCC	132	5	$\dfrac{(5\times100)}{132}=3.79\%$
217	Cardiac valve & oth maj cardiothoracic proc w card cath w CC	201	3	$\dfrac{(3\times100)}{201}=1.49\%$
239	Amputation for circ sys disorders exc upper limb & toe w MCC	8	3	$\dfrac{(3\times100)}{8}=37.50\%$
469	Major joint replacement or reattachment of lower extremity w MCC	132	4	$\dfrac{(4\times100)}{132}=3.03\%$
	Total	**819**	**30**	$\dfrac{(30\times100)}{819}=3.66\%$

Exercise 6.9

General anesthesia death rate:

$$\frac{(2 \times 100)}{663} = 0.30\%$$

Regional anesthesia death rate:

$$\frac{(1 \times 100)}{530} = 0.19\%$$

Local anesthesia death rate:

$$\frac{(1 \times 100)}{133} = 0.75\%$$

Exercise 6.11

$$\frac{(2 \times 100)}{134} = 1.49\%$$

Exercise 6.13

The **maternal mortality ratio** is the number of maternal deaths during a given period over the number of live births in a given period. (This is different from the maternal mortality rate.)

ANSWER: 10.63 rounded to 11 per 100,000

$$\frac{(440 \times 100,000)}{4,138,349} = 10.63 = 11 \, \text{per} \, 100,000$$

Exercise 6.15

$$\frac{[(2+4) \times 100]}{29+2+4} = \frac{600}{35} = 17.14\%$$

Exercise 6.17

Community Hospital
Cancer Registry Annual Report
Selected Cancer Deaths Reported
20XX

Type of Cancer	No. of Discharges	No. of Deaths	Death Rate
Prostate	23	6	$\frac{(6 \times 100)}{23} = 26.09\%$
Breast	56	4	$\frac{(4 \times 100)}{56} = 7.14\%$
Lung and Bronchus	28	9	$\frac{(9 \times 100)}{28} = 32.14\%$

Colon/Rectum	39	2	$\dfrac{(2 \times 100)}{39} = 5.13\%$
Uterus	36	5	$\dfrac{(5 \times 100)}{36} = 13.89\%$
Urinary Bladder	15	2	$\dfrac{(2 \times 100)}{15} = 13.33\%$
Non-Hodgkin's Lymphoma	21	6	$\dfrac{(6 \times 100)}{21} = 28.57\%$
Melanoma of the Skin	23	5	$\dfrac{(5 \times 100)}{23} = 21.74\%$
Kidney and Renal Pelvis	15	3	$\dfrac{(3 \times 100)}{15} = 20.00\%$
Ovary	12	5	$\dfrac{(5 \times 100)}{12} = 41.67\%$
Total	**268**	**47**	$\dfrac{(47 \times 100)}{268} = 17.54\%$

Chapter 7

Exercise 7.1
False, the calculation is
$$\frac{(6 \times 100)}{24} = 25.00\%$$

Exercise 7.3
Gross death rate:
$$\frac{(288 \times 100)}{16,523} = 1.74\%$$

Gross autopsy rate:
$$\frac{(185 \times 100)}{288} = 64.24\%$$

Net autopsy rate:
$$\frac{(185 \times 100)}{(288 - 20)} = \frac{18,500}{268} = 69.03\%$$

Exercise 7.5

Answer: **54.55%**

$$\frac{18 \times 100}{33} = 54.545 = 54.55\%$$

EXPLANATION: There were 27 inpatient deaths and 11 were autopsied. Two of the 27 deaths were coroner's cases. One of those coroner's cases was autopsied by the hospital pathologist SO IT IS COUNTED IN THE 11. Three former patients died in the ER, two former patients died in an SNF, one former patient died at home, and one died in the OP department. Add up the deaths. There were 27 inpatient deaths, but you can only count 26 because the coroner had two cases and took one and left the other for the hospital pathologists, so the one that was left can be counted in the deaths.

Exercise 7.7

Adjusted hospital autopsy rate:

36.36%

Exercise 7.9

Newborn death rate:

0.75%

The newborn death rate is the total deaths multiplied by 100 and divided by the total discharges.

$$\frac{(3 \times 100)}{398} = 0.75\%$$

Newborn autopsy rate:

66.67%

The newborn autopsy rate is the total autopsies multiplied by 100 and divided by the total deaths.

$$\frac{(2 \times 100)}{3} = 66.67\%$$

Exercise 7.11

Newborn death rate:

0.83%

The newborn death rate is the total deaths multiplied by 100 and divided by the total discharges.

$$\frac{(4 \times 100)}{483} = 0.83\%$$

Newborn autopsy rate:

50.00%

The newborn autopsy rate is the total autopsies multiplied by 100 and divided by the total deaths.

$$\frac{(2 \times 100)}{4} = 50.00\%$$

Stillbirths are not included in this formula nor are the two newborns born outside the hospital who were admitted later and died. They would be considered pediatric deaths.

Exercise 7.13

Urban Hospital

Newborn death rate:

0.84%

The newborn death rate is the 2 newborn deaths multiplied by 100 and divided by the 239 newborn discharges.

$$\frac{(2 \times 100)}{239} = 0.84\%$$

Fetal death rate:

2.04%

The fetal death rate is the 5 intermediate and late fetal deaths multiplied by 100 and divided by the sum of 240 births and 5 intermediate and late fetal deaths.

$$\frac{[(3+2) \times 100]}{[240 + (3+2)]} = \frac{500}{245} = 2.04\%$$

Newborn autopsy rate:

50.00%

The newborn autopsy rate is the 1 newborn autopsy multiplied by 100 and divided by the 2 newborn deaths.

$$\frac{(1 \times 100)}{2} = 50.00\%$$

Fetal autopsy rate:

40.00%

The fetal autopsy rate is the 2 fetal autopsies multiplied by 100 and divided by the 5 intermediate and late fetal deaths.

$$\frac{(2 \times 100)}{(3+2)} = 40.00\%$$

Exercise 7.13 (*continued*)

Suburban Hospital

Newborn death rate:

0.43%

$$\frac{(1 \times 100)}{230} = 0.43\%$$

Fetal death rate:

1.67%

$$\frac{[(3+1) \times 100]}{[235 + (3+1)]} = \frac{400}{239} = 1.67\%$$

Newborn autopsy rate:

0%
0 autopsies = 0%

Fetal autopsy rate:

25.00%

$$\frac{(1 \times 100)}{(3+1)} = 25.00\%$$

Rural Hospital

Newborn death rate:

1.23%

$$\frac{(2 \times 100)}{162} = 1.23\%$$

Fetal death rate:

1.20%

$$\frac{[(1+1) \times 100]}{[165 + (1+1)]} = \frac{200}{167} = 1.20\%$$

Newborn autopsy rate:

50.00%

$$\frac{(1 \times 100)}{2} = 50.00\%$$

Fetal autopsy rate:

100.00%

$$\frac{(2 \times 100)}{(1+1)} = 100.00\%$$

Specialty Hospital

Newborn death rate:

8.21%

$$\frac{(16 \times 100)}{195} = 8.21\%$$

Fetal death rate:

5.26%

$$\frac{[(6+5) \times 100]}{[198+(6+5)]} = \frac{1{,}100}{209} = 5.26\%$$

Newborn autopsy rate:

37.50%

$$\frac{(6 \times 100)}{16} = 37.50\%$$

Fetal autopsy rate:

63.64%

$$\frac{(7 \times 100)}{(6+5)} = 63.64\%$$

SYSTEM AS A WHOLE

Newborn death rate:

2.54%

$$\frac{(21 \times 100)}{826} = 2.54\%$$

Fetal death rate:

2.56%

$$\frac{[(13+9) \times 100]}{[838+(13+9)]} = 2.56\%$$

Newborn autopsy rate:

38.10%

$$\frac{(8 \times 100)}{21} = 38.10\%$$

Fetal autopsy rate:

54.55%

$$\frac{(12 \times 100)}{(13+9)} = 54.55\%$$

Chapter 8

Exercise 8.1

Nosocomial infection rate for adults and children:

$$\frac{(13 \times 100)}{1,784} = 0.73\%$$

Nosocomial infection rate for newborns:

$$\frac{(3 \times 100)}{123} = 2.44\%$$

Total nosocomial infection rate for the hospital:

$$\frac{[(13 + 3) \times 100]}{(1,784 + 123)} = \frac{1,300}{1,907} = 0.68\%$$

Gross death rate for this annual period:

$$\frac{[(12 + 1) \times 100]}{(1,784 + 123)} = \frac{1,300}{1,907} = 0.68\%$$

Exercise 8.3

Postoperative infection rate:

$$\frac{(12 \times 100)}{2,059} = 0.58\%$$

Postoperative death rate:

$$\frac{(10 \times 100)}{2,053} = 0.49\%$$

Exercise 8.5

Based on the information in the table below for Community Hospital, calculate (round to two decimal places) the complication rate for each service and the total for this semiannual period.

Community Hospital
Statistics
July–December 20XX

Service	Discharges	Complications	Complication Rate
Medicine	1,742	142	**8.15%**
Surgery	1,080	180	**16.67%**
Obstetrics	389	3	**0.77%**
Newborn	390	1	**0.26%**
Total	**3,601**	**326**	**9.05%**

Exercise 8.7

C-section rate:
18.49%

Newborn death rate:
0.67%

Fetal death rate:
4.03%

Exercise 8.9

Community Hospital
Surgery Service
Annual Statistics 20XX

Month	Discharges	Deaths	Consultations	Consultation Rate	Gross Death Rate
January	576	17	115	$\dfrac{(115 \times 100)}{576} = 19.97\%$	$\dfrac{(17 \times 100)}{576} = 2.95\%$
February	589	12	102	$\dfrac{(102 \times 100)}{589} = 17.32\%$	$\dfrac{(12 \times 100)}{589} = 2.04\%$
March	601	15	84	$\dfrac{(84 \times 100)}{601} = 13.98\%$	$\dfrac{(15 \times 100)}{601} = 2.50\%$
April	542	13	63	$\dfrac{(63 \times 100)}{542} = 11.62\%$	$\dfrac{(13 \times 100)}{542} = 2.40\%$
May	614	6	96	$\dfrac{(96 \times 100)}{614} = 15.64\%$	$\dfrac{(6 \times 100)}{614} = 0.98\%$
June	574	14	85	$\dfrac{(85 \times 100)}{574} = 14.81\%$	$\dfrac{(14 \times 100)}{574} = 2.44\%$
July	563	10	74	$\dfrac{(74 \times 100)}{563} = 13.14\%$	$\dfrac{(10 \times 100)}{563} = 1.78\%$
August	555	9	69	$\dfrac{(69 \times 100)}{555} = 12.43\%$	$\dfrac{(9 \times 100)}{555} = 1.62\%$
September	603	6	78	$\dfrac{(78 \times 100)}{603} = 12.94\%$	$\dfrac{(6 \times 100)}{603} = 1.00\%$

Exercise 8.9 (*continued*)

Month	Discharges	Deaths	Consultations	Consultation Rate	Gross Death Rate
October	591	7	45	$\frac{(45 \times 100)}{591} = 7.61\%$	$\frac{(7 \times 100)}{591} = 1.18\%$
November	583	5	86	$\frac{(86 \times 100)}{583} = 14.75\%$	$\frac{(5 \times 100)}{583} = 0.86\%$
December	562	12	73	$\frac{(73 \times 100)}{562} = 12.99\%$	$\frac{(12 \times 100)}{562} = 2.14\%$
Total	**6,953**	**126**	**970**	$\frac{(970 \times 100)}{6,953} = 13.95\%$	$\frac{(126 \times 100)}{6,953} = 1.81\%$

Exercise 8.11

**Community Medical Center
Annual Statistics, 20XX**

Discharges (includes deaths)	Deaths	No. of Patients Readmitted	Readmission Rate
9,305	440	903	**10.19%**

ANSWER: 10.19%

**Community Meadows Medical Center
Annual Statistics, 20XX**

Discharges (includes deaths)	Deaths	No. of Patients Readmitted	Readmission Rate
8,870	501	672	**8.03%**

ANSWER: 8.03%

Exercise 8.13

**Community Hospital
Semiannual Statistics
July–December 20XX**

Month	No. of Discharges	No. of Accounts Turned Over to a Collection Agency	Rate of Accounts Turned Over to a Collection Agency
July	302	25	$\dfrac{(25 \times 100)}{302} = 8.28\%$
August	326	30	$\dfrac{(30 \times 100)}{326} = 9.20\%$
September	342	32	$\dfrac{(32 \times 100)}{342} = 9.36\%$
October	318	15	$\dfrac{(15 \times 100)}{318} = 4.72\%$
November	352	24	$\dfrac{(24 \times 100)}{352} = 6.82\%$
December	312	19	$\dfrac{(19 \times 100)}{312} = 6.09\%$
Total	**1,952**	**145**	$\dfrac{(145 \times 100)}{1,952} = 7.43\%$

Chapter 9

Exercise 9.1

1. Total annual compensation/Total annual productivity

$$\frac{\$27{,}040}{213{,}000} = 0.087 = 0.09 \text{ or } 9 \text{ cents per line}$$

2. $$\frac{\$24{,}960}{234{,}000} = 0.106 = 0.11 \text{ or } 11 \text{ cents per line}$$

3. a. Transcriptionist who produces 1,000 lines per day at $12.00 per hour:

$$\frac{\$24{,}960}{260{,}000} = 0.096 \text{ or } 10 \text{ cents per line}$$

   Transcriptionist who produces 1,200 lines per day:

$$\frac{\$24{,}960}{312{,}000} = 0.08 = 8 \text{ cents per line}$$

   b. Both make $12.00 per hour, but one produces 1,000 and one produces 1,200 lines per day. As the production increases, the labor unit cost decreases.

   c. Transcriptionist who produces 1,000 per day at $15.00 per hour:

$$\frac{\$31{,}200}{260{,}000} = 0.12 \text{ or } 12 \text{ cents per line}$$

   Transcriptionist who produces 1,100 per day at $13.00 per hour:

$$\frac{\$27{,}040}{286{,}000} = 0.09 \text{ or } 9 \text{ cents per line}$$

   d. Total compensation/Total productivity

   The total annual salaries for the eight transcriptionists = $219,440.

   The total medical transcriptionist's annual productivity = 2,184,000 lines per year.

   The unit cost = $219,440/2,184,000 = 0.100 or 10 cents per line.

Exercise 9.3

1. Postage: $$\frac{\$465}{542} = \$0.84 \text{ per request}$$

   Service contract: $$\frac{\$216}{542} = 0.398 = \$0.40 \text{ per request}$$

Equipment: $\dfrac{\$135}{542} = 0.249 = \$0.25$ per request

Supplies: $\dfrac{\$110}{542} = \$0.20$ per request

Wages: $\$13.00 \times 2{,}080 = \$27{,}040$ per year

$\dfrac{\$27{,}040}{12} = \$2{,}253.33$ per month

$\dfrac{\$2{,}253.33}{542} = 4.157 = \$4.16$

2. Monthly cost: $\$0.84 + \$0.40 + \$0.25 + \$0.20 + \$4.16 = \$5.85$ per request $\times\ 542$ requests $= \$3{,}170.70$

3. $\$1{,}800.00 - \$3{,}170.70 = -\$1{,}370.70$

Exercise 9.5

Telephone requests: $\$3.75 \times 150 = \$562.50$

Online appointment request form: $\$150.00 \times 150 = \$225.00$

Cost savings: $\$562.50 - \$225.00 = \$337.50/150$ or $\$2.25$ per appointment

Exercise 9.7

Department	Week #1	Week #2	Week #3	Week #4	Total	Proportion
Lab	27	34	48	54	163	0.27
Radiology	15	21	26	42	104	0.17
Pathology	25	26	28	31	110	0.18
Nursing	17	22	36	41	116	0.19
Physical therapy	5	4	2	12	23	0.04
Miscellaneous	20	21	22	26	89	0.15
Total	**109**	**128**	**162**	**206**	**605**	**1.00**

Example: $\dfrac{163}{605} = 0.269 = 0.27$

Exercise 9.9

1. 5,000 inpatient records × 30 pages = 150,000

   2,000 outpatient records × 4 pages = 8,000

   1,000 ED records × 4 = 4,000

   $$\frac{(150,000+8,000+4,000)}{1,500}=108.0 \text{ days}$$

2. **ANSWER :** 3.6 FTEs needed

   $$\frac{108}{30}=3.6 \text{ FTEs}$$

   or

   $$\frac{162,000}{30}=5,400 \text{ pages needing to be scanned}$$

   $$\frac{5,400}{1,500}=3.6 \text{ FTEs}$$

3. a. Coder A: $\frac{(425\times100)}{1,300}=32.69\%$

   Coder B: $\frac{(502\times100)}{1,300}=38.62\%$

   Coder C: $\frac{(373\times100)}{1,300}=28.69\%$

   b. Coder A: $\frac{425}{21}=20.24$

   Coder B: $\frac{502}{21}=23.90$

   Coder C: $\frac{373}{21}=17.76$

   c. Coder A: $\frac{20.24}{8}=2.53$

   Coder B: $\frac{23.90}{8}=2.99$

   Coder C: $\frac{17.76}{8}=2.22$

d. Coder A: $\dfrac{60}{2.53} = 23.72$

Coder B: $\dfrac{60}{2.99} = 20.07$

Coder C: $\dfrac{60}{2.22} = 27.03$

e. Coder A: $\dfrac{(4 \times 100)}{425} = 0.94\%$

Coder B: $\dfrac{(3 \times 100)}{502} = 0.60\%$

Coder C: $\dfrac{(11 \times 100)}{373} = 2.95\%$

Exercise 9.11

1. **8 years** $\dfrac{\$28,000}{\$3,500} = 8$

In this case, the department should not purchase this equipment because the savings do not justify its purchase.

2. **22.6%**

$\$76,000 - \$62,000 = \$14,000$

$\dfrac{(\$14,000 \times 100)}{\$62,000} = 22.58 = 22.6\%$

The budget variance is the difference between actual cost and expected cost, multiplied by 100 and then divided by the expected cost.

Exercise 9.13

1. Using Worksheet No. 1 in exercise 3.9, create a computerized spreadsheet to calculate the patient census.

	12:01 a.m. Census		Adm		Trf	Total		Disch		Trf	11:59 p.m. Census			Serv days	
Day	A/C	NB	A/C	Bir	in	A/C	NB	A/C	NB	out	A/C	NB	A/D	A/C	NB
1	162	2	22	1	10	194	3	19	0	10	165	3	1	166	3
2	165	3	29	0	8	202	3	23	1	8	171	2	0	171	2
3	171	2	14	2	3	188	4	24	0	3	161	4	1	162	4
4	161	4	24	0	5	190	4	25	0	5	160	4	0	160	4
5	160	4	11	1	6	177	5	25	2	6	146	3	0	146	3
6	146	3	20	0	1	167	3	16	0	1	150	3	0	150	3
7	150	3	29	0	10	189	3	17	0	10	162	3	0	162	3
8	162	3	24	2	13	199	5	20	0	13	166	5	3	169	5
9	166	5	23	1	7	196	6	22	1	7	167	5	1	159	5
10	167	5	19	0	10	196	5	17	0	10	169	5	0	150	5
11	169	5	11	0	5	185	5	22	3	5	158	2	1	143	2
12	158	2	16	0	6	180	2	24	0	6	150	2	0	153	2
13	150	2	18	1	5	173	3	25	0	5	143	3	0	159	3
14	143	3	29	0	5	177	3	19	0	5	153	3	0	153	3
15	153	3	28	0	8	189	3	22	2	8	159	1	1	160	1
16	159	1	26	3	6	191	4	19	0	6	166	4	0	166	4
17	166	4	26	0	7	199	4	19	2	7	173	2	0	173	2
18	173	2	18	0	10	201	2	25	0	10	166	2	0	166	2
19	166	2	12	0	6	184	2	33	0	6	145	2	0	145	2
20	145	2	22	1	8	175	3	16	3	8	151	0	1	152	0
21	151	0	26	0	3	180	0	17	0	3	160	0	1	161	0
22	160	0	32	2	11	203	2	25	0	11	167	2	1	168	5
23	167	2	29	2	14	210	4	27	0	14	169	4	0	169	4
24	169	4	22	0	10	201	4	21	2	10	170	2	0	170	2
25	170	2	20	3	13	203	5	34	0	13	156	5	0	156	5
26	156	5	14	0	6	176	5	37	1	6	133	4	1	134	4
27	133	4	23	0	5	161	4	16	0	5	140	4	0	140	4
28	140	4	26	2	4	170	6	18	2	4	148	4	0	148	4
29	148	4	17	0	6	171	4	22	1	6	143	3	1	144	3
30	143	3	19	0	7	169	3	21	1	7	141	2	0	141	2
31	141	2	21	1	12	174	3	16	0	12	146	3	1	147	3
Total	4,870	90	670	22	230	5,770	112	686	21	230	4,854	91	14	4,868	91

Monthly Compilation of Inpatient Census and Inpatient Service Days — May 20XX

2. Using the table in exercise 5.4, which lists 15 patients by name, age, clinical service, and LOS, create a computerized spreadsheet to calculate the ALOS.

**Community Hospital
Discharge List
September 20, 20XX**

Pt. Name	Age	Clinical Service	Admission Date	Length of Stay
Anderson	72	Medicine	9/18	2
Bretz	43	Surgery	8/19	32
Clemments	32	Obstetrics	9/18	2
Dimmick	25	Obstetrics	9/18	2
Erichson	98	Medicine	9/1	19
Frye	67	Medicine	8/12	39
Grell	43	Surgery	9/2	18
Hallbauer	15	Obstetrics	9/19	1
Imel	33	Medicine	9/17	3
Jordan	51	Medicine	9/16	4
Kirkpatrick	23	Obstetrics	9/17	3
Locke	57	Surgery	8/3	48
Miller	48	Surgery	8/31	20
Nickel	59	Medicine	9/4	16
Oller	63	Medicine	9/9	11
Total				220
Average LOS				**14.7**

Chapter 10

Exercise 10.1

1. True

2. 27, 35, 54, 56, 65, 74, 75, 76, 77, 84, 86, 88, 89, 91, 92, 93, 94, 95, 96, 97, 99, 100

$$\frac{(11 \times 100)}{22} = 50\text{th percentile}$$

Exercise 10.3

1. The range for the data may be expressed as 17 (the difference) or as 1 to 18 (quoting the smallest and largest values); however, keep in mind that in mathematics, the range is usually expressed as one value.

Exercise 10.3 (*continued*)

    2. a. 3 to 15 or 12

         b. −4 to 15 or 19

         c. 42 to 127 or 85

    3. 3 + 22 = 25

    4. 107 − 54 = 53

    5. 227 − 127 = 100

Chapter 11

Exercise 11.1

1. This is an example of the nominal data or scale. In the nominal scale of measurement, you are only allowed to examine whether the data are equal to some particular value or to count the number of occurrences of each value. For example, gender is a nominal scale variable. You can examine whether the gender of a person is female or count the number of males in a sample.

2. This is an example of ordinal scale. Ordinal data are types of data in which the values are in ordered categories. On the ordinal scale, the order of the numbers is meaningful, not the number itself. This is because the intervals or distance between categories are not necessarily equal.

3. No, because temperature is an interval scale of measurement and the zero on the scale does not represent the absence of the thing being measured. Interval measurement ratios do not make sense: 80 degrees is not twice as hot as 40 degrees (although the attribute value is twice as large).

4. Yes, because this is an example of ratio scale of measurement. There is a zero point; that is, you can have zero patients.

5. This is an example of an ordinal scale of measurement. Measurements with ordinal scales are ordered in the sense that higher numbers represent higher values. However, the intervals between the numbers are not necessarily equal. For example, on the 5-point rating scale measuring correct information given by the clerk, the difference between a rating of 2 and a rating of 3 may not represent the same difference as the difference between a rating of 4 and a rating of 5.

6. The scales of these variables would be: **b. nominal, ratio, ordinal, ordinal.** The first question, whether the mothers drank, is answered yes or no. In the nominal scale, observations are organized into categories. The birth weight of the baby is a ratio scale, which has a defined unit of measure, a real zero point, and equal intervals between successive values. The Apgar scores at one minute and at five minutes are examples of ordinal data.

Exercise 11.3

Community Hospital
Ages of Patients with Colon Cancer
Annual Statistics, 20XX

Age	No. of Patients	Proportion
≤ 30	3	**0.01**
31–40	12	**0.06**
41–50	18	**0.09**
51–60	60	**0.29**
61–70	65	**0.32**
71+	48	**0.23**
Total patients	206	

For example, the proportion of ages less than or equal to 30 is the number of patients in that category divided by the total number of patients (206).

Example: $\dfrac{3}{206} = 0.014 = 0.01$

Exercise 11.5

Analyze the report, then prepare the data displays indicated in the list below. The data displays may be neatly hand drawn or created using a software program.

1. Create a histogram to display the distribution of total days by age.

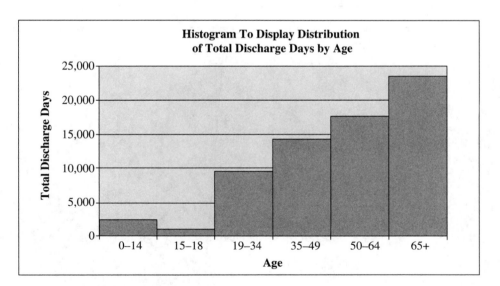

Exercise 11.5 (*continued*)

2. Create a bar graph to display the admission by day of week for Medicare patients in comparison to the admission by day of week for all patients.

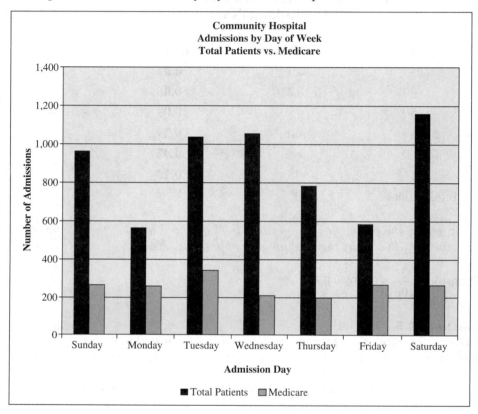

3. Create a pie chart to display the percentage of patients discharged by major service category.

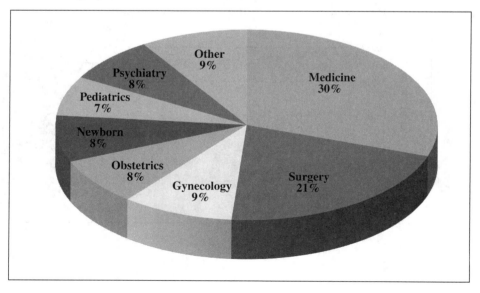

4. Create a table for length of stay distribution.

LENGTH OF STAY DISTRIBUTION

	PATIENTS	% CASES
SAME DAY	114	1.7
1 DAY	755	11.3
2–4 DAYS	1,343	20.2
5–7 DAYS	1,555	23.3
8–14 DAYS	1,469	22.0
15–42 DAYS	1,217	18.3
43+ DAYS	210	3.2
Total	6,663	100.0

Exercise 11.7

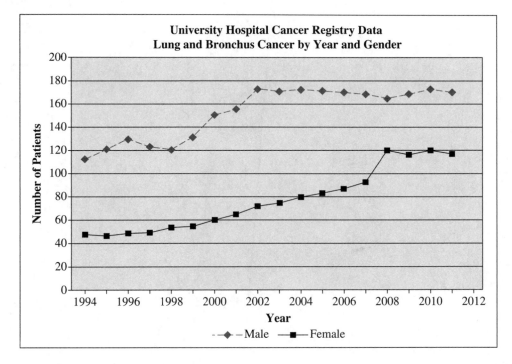

Chapter 12

Exercise 12.1

Order	Description
5	Analyze the data
3	Design the research
1	Define the problem
6	Draw conclusions
2	Review the literature
4	Collect the data

Chapter 13

Exercise 13.1

Fail to reject the null hypothesis, or not statistically significant at the 0.05 level. This is because there is a greater than 5% chance that the null hypothesis is correct.

Index

Abortion, death after, 82, 83
Accidental death, 81, 82
Accreditation agencies
    reporting C-section rates to, 124
    as users of health statistics, 6
Adjusted hospital autopsy rate
    definition of, 101
    example of, 101
    formula for calculating, 101
Admission and discharge, same-day, 27,
        31, 32
Admission date, 58
    subtracted from discharge date to find
        LOS, 59
Admissions and discharges (A&Ds), 58
ADT system, complete master census and, 24
Alternative hypothesis, 232
Ambulatory care facilities, 4
    calculating length of time spent in, 60
    census of, 4
American Medical Association (AMA), reporting
        C-section rates to, 124
American Statistical Association, 244
Analysis of variance (ANOVA), 242, 255–56
Anesthesia, major types of, 80
Anesthesia death rate
    definition of, 80
    formula for calculating, 80
Annual productivity
    examples of, 138–39
    formula for, 138
ANOVA (analysis of variance), 242, 255–56
Antepartum deaths, 82
Applied research, definition of, 228
Audits of work output, 148
Autopsies, hospital, 99–100
Autopsy, 96

Autopsy rate, 95–113
    vs. death rates, 96
    definition of, 96
    fetal, 105
    gross, 96–97
    hospital, 99–101
    net, 97–98
    newborn, 104
    size of, 96
Average
    definition of, 20
    formula for, 20
Average daily inpatient census, 38–39
    formula for, 38
    for patient care unit, 39
Average daily newborn census, formula for, 39
Average duration of hospitalization, 63. *See also*
        Average length of stay (ALOS)
Average length of stay (ALOS)
    avoiding distortions in calculating, 177
    decreasing, trend toward, 63
    definition of, 63
    for financial reporting of MS-DRGs, 58
    formula for, 63
    measures of central tendency used in, 175
    median used to compute, 177, 178
    sample reports for, 156–57
    verifying, with computerized discharge
        reports, 155
Average newborn length of stay
    calculating, 64, 65
    formula for, 64

Bar chart. *See* Bar graph or chart
Bar graph or chart, 207–10
    one-variable, 207, 208
    overview of, 207

Length of stay (LOS) (*continued*)
  sample calculation of, 59
  skewness in, 188
  uses of data for, 58
  variance in, 183–84, 186
Likert scale, 197
Line graphs, 212
  to display data over time, 212
  one-variable, 207, 213
  scale captions on, 206–7
  two-variable, 214
  x- and y-axis labels for, 212
Literature review for research, 230
Long-term care facilities, leave of absence for, 27
Loose papers, as labor unit cost, 143

Managed care organizations (MCOs), 6
  as users of health statistics, 6
Maternal death, definition of, 81
Maternal death rate, 81–82
  formula for calculating, 82, 85
  vital statistics computed for, 82–83
Mathematical expressions, 10–20
Mathematics review, 9–22
Mean, 2
  definition of, 175
  less dispersion around, 184
  as measure of central tendency, 176
  as preferable measure in statistical analyses, 179–80
  sensitivity to outliers of, 176, 177
  squared deviations of, 183
  standard error of, 250–51
  sum of deviations from, 184
  symbol for, 20, 176
  tests of, 250–56
Measurements, normal distribution of data, 185
Measures of central tendency, 175–80
Measures of variance, 181
Median
  calculation of, 176
  definition of, 176
  example of, 177
  use in ALOS calculation, 177, 178
  use of, to represent series, 180
Medical examiner (ME), 98
Medicare-severity diagnosis-related group (MS-DRG), ALOS to compare patients in, 58
Medication data software, 242
Mental health facilities as users of health statistics, 6
Military time, 60
Mode
  in bimodal or multimodal distributions, 179
  definition of, 178
  used when typical value is preferable, 180

Morbidity, 116
Morbidity rates, 115–35
Morgue, 96
Mortality data, 72
Mortality data report, CMS, 72
Mortality rates. *See also* Death rates
  cancer, 90–91
  definition of, 90
  neonatal and infant, 86
  newborn, 85–86
  vital statistics formula for, 82
Multimodal distribution curve, 189

Narrative reports, 224
National Center for Health Statistics (NCHS) of CDC, 4–5, 90
National Healthcare Safety Network (NHSN), 116
National Nosocomial Infections Surveillance (NNIS) System, 116, 121
National Surveillance System for Healthcare Workers (NaSH), 116
National Vital Statistics System (NVSS), 4
Naturalistic observation, 233
Necropsy, 96
Negative skew, 188
Neonatal death, 85
Neonatal mortality rate formula, 86
Net autopsy rate
  definition of, 97
  example of, 98
  formula for calculating, 98
  vs. gross autopsy rate, 98
Net death rate, 75–76
  definition of, 75
  example of, 76
  formula for calculating, 76
Newborn autopsy rate
  definition of, 104
  example of, 104
  formula for calculating, 104
Newborn bassinet count, 44
Newborn bassinet occupancy ratio
  example of, 52
  formula for, 51
Newborn census, 32, 38–39
  average daily, 39
Newborn death, 85
  rates, formula for calculating, 86
Newborn inpatients, gross death rate and, 73
Newborn mortality rates, 85–86
  definitions for, 85
  formula for calculating, 86
Newborn vs. pediatric admission, 105
Nominal, definition of, 196
Nominal data, 196